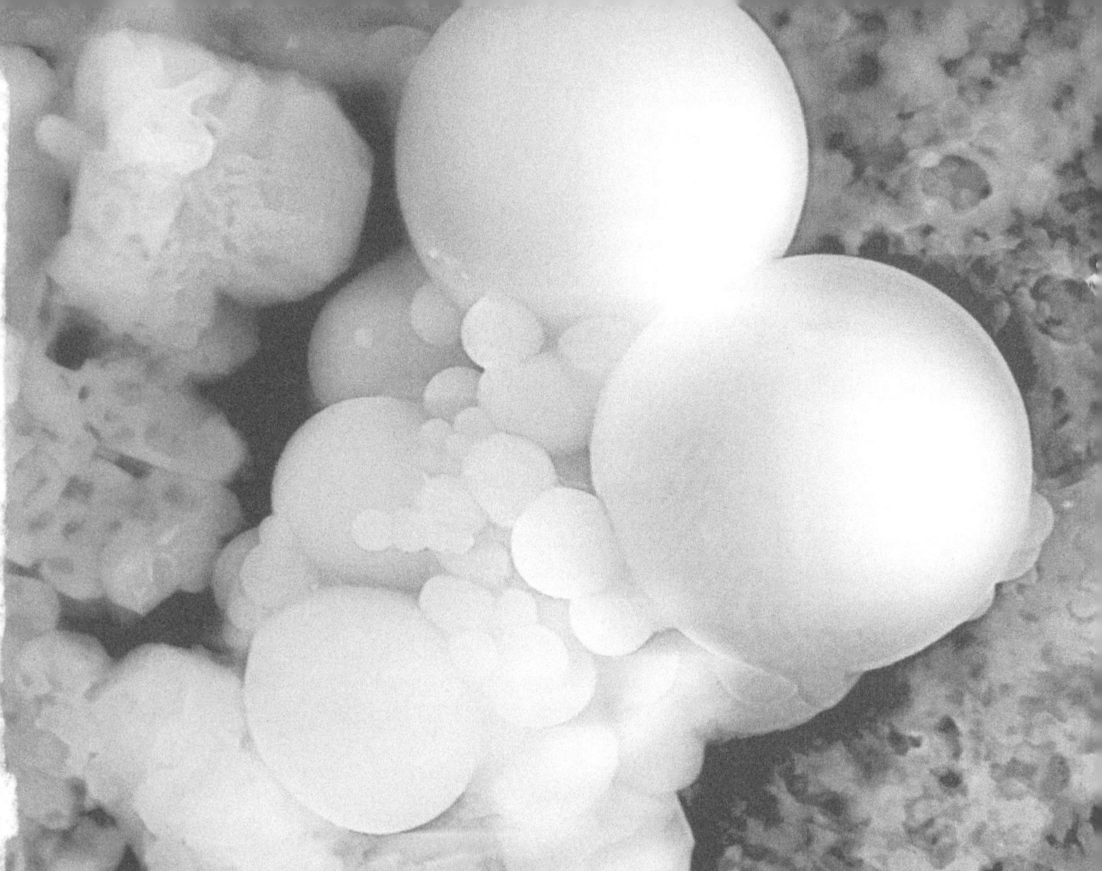

Advances in Nanopathology

Advances in Nanopathology
From Vaccines to Food

Antonietta Morena Gatti
Stefano Montanari

JENNY STANFORD
PUBLISHING

Published by

Jenny Stanford Publishing Pte. Ltd.
Level 34, Centennial Tower
3 Temasek Avenue
Singapore 039190

Email: editorial@jennystanford.com
Web: www.jennystanford.com

British Library Cataloguing-in-Publication Data
A catalogue record for this book is available from the British Library.

Advances in Nanopathology: From Vaccines to Food

ISBN 978-981-4877-29-9 (Hardcover)
ISBN 978-1-003-05622-5 (eBook)

This book is dedicated to man, his stupidity and the sword of Damocles, which he himself hung on his head.

In fact, man is the only animal living on this planet who is busy building the tools of his own death.

Contents

Preface

Though this book was written for the benefit of our students, we dare to be presumptuous enough to believe that it can be useful for many other categories of readers. For example, politicians and policymakers with something to do with public health and environment, chemists, physicists, biologists, pharmacists, engineers and, above all, medical doctors. But, unfortunately, this last category is the most difficult to approach and the most impervious. Nowadays, it is imperative that they know the basic concepts that will be exposed in the chapters of this book, as they are fundamental to the work they are called upon to do. If observed from an objective, epistemological standpoint, medicine is not a science. At least, not a science in its own right. Among others, the most important key feature missing is repeatability, and this makes the doctor's job extremely difficult. Therefore, they need a great erudition, elasticity of mind, intelligence and honesty, wise humility included: something that, in truth, is not always the case. Doctors are not scientists, but every day they are called upon to use the results of scientific research. For that reason they must keep themselves updated, must be able to distinguish what is really worth extricating among a huge amount of a literature of which it would be prudent to doubt and even less reliable news, and use the data exclusively in the interest of their patients according to the often referred to but not always kept the Hippocratic oath and the dictates of modern bioethics.

Hospitals and private practices are crowded with patients. In some circumstances, cases are urgent, and decisions should be taken in a matter of a few minutes. So, of course with some exceptions, doctors rely on shortcuts, often in the form of more or less official guidelines, that is, a means to reach diagnoses and therapies that are nothing more than one-size-fits-all, a series of steps prepared by agencies midway between medicine and bureaucracy, something that will never fit any human organism in all their personal, unrepeatable, unique, ever-changeable varieties, as many as there are human beings. Uncertain as they are, shortcuts have at least two advantages: they are quick and they exempt the doctor from many legal responsibilities, a feature that is gaining more and more importance. And in many cases, they work with the help as essential as disowned of homeostasis, that is, the natural tendency of any organism to maintain or regain its internal stability: in a word, its health. 'Most patients will heal in spite of your treatment' is what one of our teachers of yore used to tell us students.

It's obvious: The planet teems with sick people, and it's impossible to reserve the due time and the due attention to each of them. Then, to make things more complicated, there are many other factors influencing the treatment of those subjects: the insufficient knowledge achieved by science and medicine (e.g., we still have thousands of so-called orphan diseases and the number doesn't show signs of dwindling), law and litigations, the interference of pharmaceutical and medical-devices industry, the censorship put in place by medical journals, a problem, this, denounced by important people involved in the work but in fact ignored.

To be effective, medicine must be tailored for each subject. That's nobody's fault or responsibility: Nature wanted the human body to be terribly complicated and open to infinite variables. So, though willy-nilly, if we, doctors included, want to be effective, we have no other choice but to come to terms with the situation. We are perfectly aware of the fact: in most cases tailoring is too hard to do or actually impossible to put into practice, so medicine resorts to simplifications. Too often to oversimplifications.

To be effective, medicine must start from a correct, full understanding of the problem, but when particulate pollution is concerned – that is, the subject we deal with – we see too many wrong diagnoses. It is only obvious that missing a diagnosis prompts the implementation of a therapy that in some instances is ineffective, in others definitely harmful, and in any case, however one looks at the situation, precious time is lost. So, here, with this book, without absolutely falling into the naivety of presuming to substitute ourselves for doctors, we try to offer more data on which doctors can reason and make their diagnoses through which, hopefully, they can apply a suitable therapy, never forgetting the obvious: No therapy works and is as successful as not to get sick. And here come into play policymakers who must decide what kind of world we are to live in, since many pathologies, at least those that are the subject of our research, come from the environment, from what we breathe, from what we eat, from the medicines we take and even from reasons hard to suspect like, for instance and among other things, from what we wear or even from how we wash our laundry or freshen the rooms we live in. Thus, in the manner of Plato's ideal politicians, they must act according to knowledge and conscience.

If conscience is mainly a matter of family upbringing, knowledge comes from study and, in our case, the help of specialists like chemists, physicists, biologists, pharmacists and engineers, who, in their turn, must be updated and act according to conscience.

In short, medicine must be more open and more extended, must be partially reformed and must be freed from a ballast now become too heavy and too hard to carry. The first characteristic of the new scientist and the new medical doctor, the most important, is to have their minds free from preconceptions, wherever they come from.

If doctors are of the utmost importance, scientists and technicians are probably no less. For instance, engineers are called upon to design facilities, plants and equipment, and in many circumstances they don't take into due consideration the actual consequences of what results from the use of the products they have designed and planned and the final fate of the product at its usable life's end. To them, and in particular to those who pay for the project and aim at getting as much money as possible from it, and quickly, what is important is to obtain immediate results without caring what the consequences are in terms of health and environment. As a matter of fact, in most cases no one will ask them to answer for their deed.

What we keep seeing through our analyses is an increasing pollution of the environment, of what we eat, of the drugs we take and of the products we currently use, and we detect in more and more cases particulate pollutants inside pathological tissues not only taken from adults but even from newborn babies and unborn foetuses. It is all too easy to predict that the situation will soon become extremely critical and the necessary countermeasures must be taken. Obviously, to be able to do that, the full knowledge of the situation must reach the culture of everybody, no matter if scientist, medical doctor, politician or man in the street. Journalists are also important: often newspapers, radios and TVs report news or publish considerations that are not only scientifically objectionable or false at all, but that can be in mutual conflict, ranging from the most radiant optimism to the direst pessimism. Truth does not lie simplistically in the middle but must be looked for and assessed in each case.

Finally, an important notice for those who will be patient enough to read this book. It is a usual occurrence that many of those who approach our research superficially define it as belonging to the so-called 'alternative medicine'. Nothing further from reality: What we do is science in the strictest of manners, and the part that concerns medicine is what most classically exists in its scope. Ours is just a different or, better, an additional point of view of exactly the same panorama and our only purpose is to bring to light data that, though indisputable in their validity, do not collect attention or, when they do, in most cases are misunderstood.

In these pages there will be no axioms or dogmas or anything outside of science as science must be understood, that is to say a, domain where everything is derived from observations and everything is demonstrated. Some basic concepts will be repeated on several occasions throughout the book. It was done on purpose, not to bore the reader but because students often have the habit of reviewing the various chapters separately and, in any case, so that our readers remember them and always take them into account. These are very simple concepts, yet it is not uncommon to prefer to leave them aside simply because they are not in line with what looks convenient to the *Homo sapiens* of the 21st century.

Antonietta Morena Gatti

Stefano Montanari

December 2020

Chapter 1

Introduction

1.1 How Nanopathology Was Born

At the beginning of the nineties a surgeon gave us a vena cava filter he had removed from a patient. He had done so because, for reasons he did not know but which he was curious about, that metal device had failed and had broken inside his patient's inferior vena cava.

Nowadays, in similar circumstances, nobody would cut open a subject to remove a broken filter. That particular surgery is quite challenging, and the advantage obtained, if any, is minimal indeed since that device, even if in conditions which are certainly not ideal and because of that being unable to work properly, does not cause inconveniences, at least in general. But, regardless of any consideration which does not belong to us, we got that filter along with the question 'Why did it break?'

The answer was quite easy: it had broken because it had slid caudally, and one of its six prongs had entered one of the renal veins, getting stuck there. The movement counterstream but in favour of gravity towards the iliac junction with a prong which, blocked as it was, could not follow the rest of the device, and the continuous, repeated deformations of the filter brought about by respiration and, especially, by Valsalva maneuvers had eventually caused the failure. Nothing particularly interesting: only the technical observation that the filter had been placed too cranially.

Advances in Nanopathology: From Vaccines to Food
Antonietta Morena Gatti and Stefano Montanari

ISBN 978-981-4877-29-9 (Hardcover), 978-1-003-05622-5 (eBook)
www.jennystanford.com

What was interesting and, indeed, baffling was something which had nothing to do with the original question, that is, what we found on the surface of the device and, more in particular, at the fracture point. Looking there through an electron microscope and with the aid of an instrument called energy-dispersive spectrometer (EDS), we found chemical elements which did not belong either to the filter or to the human body. Why they were there was a question we had no answer to, and somewhat sadly, it was something which did not interest the doctors we consulted.

Some months after, we faced the same problem but, in that circumstance, with a different brand of filter, made of a different metal alloy: AISI 316 L stainless steel in the former case, and Phynox, a cobalt-chromium-nickel-based alloy, in the latter. Also in that circumstance, we got the same qualitative result: chemical elements different from what we found in the first device but, again, definitely foreign both to the filter and the human body. Same question, same answer: we did not know where they could come from, and the problem, puzzling to us, did not seem to interest anybody. So, in both cases, our questions about the drugs those patients were taking because of their health conditions were greeted with some annoyance. Evidently, what can't find an immediate, credible enough or anyhow accepted explanation is removed from the brain and wondering about it is considered a waste of time.

We kept thinking that something foreign to the organism like those elements could somehow enter the blood circulation, and medicaments were the agent we suspected most, but without any evidence.

It was only at the end of 1997 that we found the answer.

After an unsuccessful tour through many hospitals, a patient had come to the University Hospital of Modena (Italy), lamenting a collection of troubles: fever for more than eight years, lachrymation from one eye, pain at the ipsilateral ear and, what was more important, liver and kidneys in a very poor condition, so that turning to a chronic hemodialysis treatment seemed inevitable.

A biopsy was taken of the liver and of the kidney, and the diagnosis issued by the histopathologist was 'cryptogenic granulomatosis of both organs'. A granulomatosis is a particular inflammatory condition of a tissue. Cryptogenic is a learned word whose meaning is nothing more than 'I do not understand why'.

The cases have already been described in a few publications, and it is not worth repeating a more accurate description than the one which can be found in our books *Nanopathology: The Health Impact of Nanoparticles* (Pan Stanford Publishing, now Jenny Stanford Publishing) and *Case Studies in Nanotoxicology and Particle Toxicology* (Elsevier Academic Press). We will limit ourselves to report that we analysed the biopsic samples of the liver and the kidney with an electron microscope equipped with an EDS and found micro- and nanoparticles made of ceramic embedded in the tissues. Those particles had behaved for what they were – foreign bodies – and, as such, had attracted macrophages which released cytokines, and an inflammatory reaction had started – hence the formation of granulomatous tissue which had caused the fever and the malfunction of the kidneys and the liver.

The origin of the ceramic particles was found in the two dental bridges the patient carried. They were badly made, and the subject, feeling uncomfortable with them, became a bruxer, thus wearing out the ceramic the prostheses were made of. To make matters worse, the dentist filed the prostheses. The small fragments had been ingested and, reasonably travelling through the circulatory system, had reached the two organs.

The solution to lachrymation and pain in the ear was easily found in replacing the two dental bridges with as many well-made ones, while fever and problems with the kidneys and the liver were palliated by administering a cortisone-based therapy, a therapeutic strategy which saved the patient from haemodialysis. It may be interesting to add that, as soon as the patient interrupted the anti-inflammatory treatment, the symptoms of the organs involved reappeared. The reason is easily explained: the micro- and nanofragments were not biodegradable, and were still there as an inflammation inducer.

Starting from the basis of that case, though with great difficulty, we started to investigate the biopsic samples of cryptogenic granulomatosis stored in hospital archives, and we noticed that in all cases, that is, when the pathology was not due to bacteria, parasites, etc., and its origin could not be found, the cause was the presence of non-degradable micro- and nanometric foreign bodies.

That successfully solved case gave us also the answer to our question about the puzzling chemical elements we had detected on the two vena cava filters we had investigated. For some reason, the subjects involved had ingested (or, as we later discovered, possibly inhaled) micro- and nanoparticles which were carried by the blood and some of them had deposited on the surface of the device they carried.

After a few very difficult years, we got a grant from the European Commission which allowed us to carry out our research (nanopathology) in a more efficient way. Then, after that first project was concluded, another European grant enabled us to get further, very important results. The project called DIPNA (FP6-NMP-STRP 032131) about nanotoxicology made us understand what the basic mechanisms of toxicity are of nanoparticles, be they engineered or accidentally produced.

1.1.1 What Is Nanopathology?

Nowadays it may sound unbelievable, but it was only at the end of the 19th century that the so-called *miasmatic theory* was abandoned by medicine. According to that universally accepted line of thinking supported, among others, by an authority as was Galen, infectious diseases, and not only those, were due to a sort of 'bad air' or miasma, a Greek word (*μίασμα*) meaning pollution. The firm belief was that particularly during the night, the soil, urban ghettoes, rotting vegetation and foul water give off noxious organic matter, causing what then were called *zymotic diseases*, those we now call infectious. Of course, there was a huge number of 'demonstrations' to back the assumption. An academic school of thought of the 1800s, somewhat extending the limits of the theory, even maintained that one could become obese just by smelling food.

That century-old theory, supported by all top 'scientists', was finally replaced, but only after having defeated a very strong resistance, by *germ theory*: infectious diseases are caused by microorganisms. It was Gerolamo Fracastoro in the mid-16th century who first intuited the phenomenon, but it was only the works of Louis Pasteur and Robert Koch which provided the irrefutable evidence with research begun in the 1850s and finally accepted, not always willingly, in the 1880s. Just to get an idea of what the scientific approach used to be, the great Rudolf Virchow (died in 1902) ridiculed Pasteur and boasted that he had never brought his eye near a microscope. One of its strong points to demonstrate how wrong Pasteur was, was, 'If microbes were responsible for illnesses, ubiquitous as they are, we were all ill.' An argument which shows an insufficient knowledge of how biology works but an argument which resurfaces again about the pathologies induced by particles.

There is no doubt: the discoveries of Pasteur and Koch gave a fundamental turning to medicine, allowing a much more correct and efficient approach to the understanding and diagnosis of many pathologies and, as a consequence, what is even more important, to the implementation of much more effective therapies.

But what they did and the impulse to research which they gave, though still lasting, is not enough. Pathologies are not only the infectious ones, and nowadays we witness the dramatic increase of diseases which once were rare when not unknown or non-existent at all. As a matter of fact, the so-called *orphan diseases*, pathologies about which we know very little and to which there are no therapies available, can be counted in several thousands. In addition, for a non-negligible number of known diseases the real cause is partially unknown, utterly ignored or, maybe and with even worse consequences, misunderstood. Unfortunately, not unlike what happened with the criticisms on miasmatic theory and many other medical beliefs, there are discoveries which, though supported by indisputable evidence, are not welcome. To this grudging reception many explanations can be put forward, from mental laziness to fear of the new, from presumption to vested interest.

We humans are an integral and inseparable part of the environment like all other animals, vegetables and any living being, and like them, we suffer the interference which we receive from what surrounds us. And dust is one interference along with heat and cold, radiations, electric and magnetic fields, humidity, noise, etc.

Human beings have always lived with dust. Volcanoes eruptions, the sand raised by the wind, rock erosion and occasional fires are all sources of natural dust. In all cases, that dust is harmful, since it can be inhaled as it floats in the atmosphere, or can be ingested when it falls on fruit, vegetables, cereals, etc., and our organism does not accept it willingly. But, for that matter, nature has a number of mechanisms to kill any creature which inhabits the planet in order to make place to new lives, and dust is one of her means. Nature has produced solid particles for billions of years, and, to that production, starting about half a million years ago, though with great geographic differences, man has started to add his own.

Every combustion generates dust, and when man discovered how to turn on the fire, a novel type of pollution appeared on the earth. Many centuries after, man learned how to use that fire, how to cook food, how to fabricate artifacts, so something unknown to nature was introduced into the environment: waste.

Nature does not have the concept of waste. What a living being discards is used as a rule by other beings for their lives. The simplest example of that is the carbon cycle, that is, the substance turnover by which carbon is exchanged among the biosphere, the soil, the water and the atmosphere of the earth. That can be easily illustrated by the physiology of the *Viridiplantae*, that is, the green plants which get most of their energy from sunlight through photosynthesis, using water and carbon dioxide. What that complicated chemical process discards is oxygen, a gas essential to the life of many animals, man included. But what those animals discard is carbon dioxide, thus restarting the cycle. Along with the nitrogen cycle and the water cycle, the carbon cycle comprises a sequence of natural events, incidentally not reproducible by man's technology, which are what makes our planet capable of sustaining life. In short, nature works in a circular way.

Man is the only being living in a linear way, which simply means living against nature's rules. As by-products of many of our activities, we introduce into the planet something which nature does not recognise and has no means to utilise. If, at the beginning of our technical progress, our technological processes were very simple and we were, after all, rare animals, now the human population has grown to exceed seven billion and, what is more critical, our technology has become extremely sophisticated, in addition to being, unfortunately, too often out of control, at least as far as its final consequences is concerned.

As it has already been mentioned, all high-temperature operations produce particles and, as a rule of thumb, those particles are the smaller, which means the more capable of creeping into the body, the higher the temperature at which they are produced. If up to not many years ago it was technically difficult and expensive to reach high temperatures, nowadays the task has become not only easy but cheap, with all the positive consequences on the possibility to make newer and cheaper products and the negative ones on the environment. So, the environment is being invaded by a growing quantity of unnatural, smaller and smaller particles, and it is those particles which are mainly responsible for the long list of diseases we, back in the late nineties, called nanopathologies.

Like it or not, these illnesses are growing more and more common and, furthermore, pathologies once unknown or, even more often, sets of diseases which apparently have nothing to do with each other are beginning to become usual.

They will be discussed in more detail later in this book, but as an anticipation, it comes to some cardiovascular diseases, cancers, neuroendocrine diseases, behaviour abnormalities, miscarriages, foetal malformations, reproduction disorders, etc.

For many years, medicine has been using histological observations performed through optical microscopy. For reasons related to the wavelength of visible light, with this system it is in fact impossible to exceed 1500 magnifications. Much more recently, molecular biology has become part of medical research. With this approach, what happens at the molecular level is evaluated without, however, having a vision of it but only getting an analytical knowledge. A very wide dimensional gap (3 to 4 orders of magnitude) opens up between the two approaches, and in that dimensional range matter behaves in a different way from that of the atom or molecule and from what exists within the dimensions visible under an optical microscope. That is precisely the gap which is filled by the electron microscopy technique which we use and which we propose.

Appendix: Deep Vein Thrombosis and Caval Filtration

In a sense, it is thanks to our interest in caval filters, deep vein thrombosis and pulmonary thrombo-embolism that nanopathology was born.

Three broad categories of factors contribute to the formation of thrombi, that is, blood clots inside a vein or an artery: hypercoagulability, an impediment to the blood flow or an excessively turbulent flow and an endothelial injury. Though Rudolf Virchow, the already mentioned German scientist of the nineteenth century, never suggested those three factors as responsible for thrombosis but saw them as a consequence of that pathology, they are grouped together under the name of *Virchow's Triad*. We will see later in this book that there is a fourth origin of blood clots, and that is the presence of micro- and nanoparticles in the blood. In that case, a nanopathology.

The formation of thrombi is a rather common occurrence in the venous system, but the majority of people have the physiological ability to dissolve them very quickly thanks to four enzyme pathways whose function is to reduce *thrombin* (a serine protease) production and/or its activity. *Plasmin* is the major enzyme of the fibrinolytic system, and its function is that of dissolving already formed clots by degrading *fibrin*.

In a minority of people or under certain circumstances like, among many others, bone fractures, long-lasting immobility in bed, major surgery, pregnancy, overweight, cancer, tobacco smoking and the use of some contraceptive drugs, there is a risk of the formation of thrombi, particularly in the veins of the lower limbs and the pelvis. That pathology is called *deep-vein thrombosis*. In general, a venous thrombus starts forming at the inner wall of the vessel (tunica intima) and grows in the direction of the heart. In some circumstances, the vein is occluded by the growing thrombus, while in others the thrombus breaks off, is carried by the bloodstream, crosses the right heart and reaches the pulmonary circulation. The phenomenon is called *pulmonary thrombo-embolism*. Since the pulmonary vessels containing venous blood (inside the lungs, they are called arteries) grow smaller and smaller in diameter, while proceeding towards the alveoli, when the thrombus arrives where the lumen is smaller than its size and is wedged there, the vessel is inevitably occluded. If the thrombus is big enough to stop the flow in a large vessel, the condition is a life-threatening one.

Anticoagulant and fibrinolytic drugs working with various mechanisms are normally used in those circumstances to try and dissolve the thrombus. When there is a danger of recurrence of thrombo-embolism, the usual prescription is that of a chronic, often life-long, therapy generally based on drugs antagonising vitamin K1 recycling, drugs initially used as pesticides against rats and mice which, ingesting them, died of internal bleeding.

The dosage of those drugs is not easy because the body's reaction to them changes rather quickly even with the ingestion of some food and the dosage needs to be frequently adjusted. There are cases where those drugs are contraindicated, often due to the risk of haemorrhage, particularly in people living an active life and, therefore, with the possibility to incur a road accident or other traumas. Although used in a minority of cases, the safest means to prevent a thrombo-embolism, then, is implanting inside the inferior vena cava, at the level of the renal veins, a filter, for some years also available in removable versions.

The models are rather numerous, and their look is quite varied, but the most common is that of six thin metal stems joined at the top of a conical shape like the framework of a tepee. Each stem has a distal hook with which the device is secured at the vein's wall.

The clot which is carried by the bloodstream towards the right heart travels along the central axis of the vessel where the speed is higher, is captured by the apex of the filter where the prongs leave the narrowest passage, is lapped by the bloodstream and more or less quickly dissolves.

There are cases in which caval filtration is ineffective, since there is no actual thrombus focus, downstream of which a filter could be reasonably placed. Patients suffering from the so-called *Trousseau's syndrome,* that is, the formation of thrombi in case of cancer or endocarditis where no consistent and identifiable origin exists, will not gain any benefit from the filter. What is interesting for our discussion is the so-called *migratory venous thrombosis,* also a condition belonging to that syndrome and the subject of uncertain explanations. We will see later in this book how, at least in certain circumstances, it can be explained.

Chapter 2

The Concept of Biocompatibility

2.1 Introduction

At the risk of being sentimentally romantic, the human body can be defined as a delicate shrine, and before introducing something into it, it is at least prudent to answer a few questions: Is the material implanted, injected or, no matter how, introduced compatible with the body? Is the whole object acceptable? Is the interaction between the foreign body and the organism components physiologically compatible? How long can it stay compatible?

When there is no sure answer, confirmed by in vitro and in vivo experiments, it is advisable not to use the product. The so-called *precautionary principle* states as much and is law in many countries, but the law is almost never applied.

The biomedical/pharmaceutical industries, but also most technologists, tend to underestimate or utterly overlook this basic, obvious concept which they consider contrary to progress.

Replacements for body parts lost through injury, amputation or disease have been in use for millennia. In 1998, some archaeologists unearthed what is believed to be the most ancient artificial eye in the world, a prosthesis made of bitumen paste dated to about 5000 years ago, discovered at the necropolis of *Shahr-i-Sokhta* in the Sistan desert on the Iran–Afghan border. A prosthetic big toe composed of leather, moulded and stained wood, and thread was discovered near

Advances in Nanopathology: From Vaccines to Food
Antonietta Morena Gatti and Stefano Montanari

ISBN 978-981-4877-29-9 (Hardcover), 978-1-003-05622-5 (eBook)
www.jennystanford.com

Luxor, belonging to a female mummy dated between 950 and 710 BC. A prosthesis which certainly was not functional but, in a certain way, was to be considered aesthetic. Then, arms, legs, dentures, even a silver nose worn by the sixteenth-century Danish astronomer Tycho Brahe (who lost his in a duel). None of them, however, was inserted into the body. For this to be done, knowledge and technologies were needed, then and for a very long time not available and, it must be admitted, even today not exactly absolutely certain.

The first 'modern' definition of biocompatibility is dated 1982.

Already at that time many prostheses were implanted in the human body to substitute an organ or part of it, to replace a tissue or to make up for a function which, for any reason, had gone lost.

Starting from years long before the eighties, probably the most common prostheses were those replacing bones or joints. A great impulse was done by the wars, since the wounds and mutilations prompted by projectiles, bombs and explosions in general caused 'not normal' lesions and orthopaedists had to 'invent' prosthetic tools, in some cases made especially for that particular case.

Most of the prostheses were manufactured according to the general indications given by an orthopaedist and were a sort of compromise between the anatomical location they were meant to occupy, the function they had to accomplish and the mechanical stresses they had to endure. Because of that, when mechanics was the main concern, it was rather customary that those materials were selected by technicians with great experience in mechanics but very little or not so great in biology, physiology and pathology. Unfortunately, then, medical doctors and surgeons had a rather primitive knowledge of materials and the final result was not particularly satisfactory.

But it was not in the field of orthopaedics alone that prostheses showed problems. For years, heart pacemakers were encapsulated in plastic materials (silicone and epoxy resins) which were prone to absorb water and swelled, a problem in some cases aggravated by their permeability to the gases leaked and released by defective batteries.

Because of wear, prosthetic heart valves lost tiny fragments of their plastic ball or of their plastic disc(s), and in other models which enjoyed a relatively short-lived popularity, they lost silver particles of the coating meant to prevent the growth of pathological tissue.

The definition of biomaterial, where the prefix 'bio' means 'compatible with a living organism', was '. . . any substance, other than a drug, or combination of substances, synthetic or natural in origin, which can be used for any period of time, as a whole or as a part of a system which treats, augments or replaces any tissue, organ or function of the body' [1].

That was a definition specifically addressed to the specific activity and supposed durability of the material in contrast with other 'similar' materials used in other fields (in cars, in architecture, etc.). The definition included the concept of temporary implant.

In 1986 the definition was enhanced, adding 'non-viable material, used in medical device, intended to interact with biological systems'. This definition opened a new scenario, since it became necessary to assess when a material is actually fit for the human body. At that time, new tests considering the interaction of the candidate materials with cells, tissues and organs started to be developed and new parameters of compatibility had to be found. Most of the tests were initially borrowed from those used by toxicologists to assess the toxicity of substances in molecular, atomic or ionic form, but when particles were understood to be toxic, and toxic in a way that is not the same as that of atoms and molecules, those tests proved to be not only useless but misleading.

One of the toxicologist's tenets, probably the main one, is Paracelsus's adage 'sola dosis facit venenum' or, a little more in detail, translating literally from his Latin, 'All things are poison and nothing is without poison. Only the dose makes a thing not a poison.' From this, the concept immediately derived is that, below a certain dose, any substance can be tolerated by the body.

All that science elaborated in the field of toxicity was verified in order to find tests and already developed standards and adapt them to biomaterials. What we want to emphasise is that atoms and molecules do not behave the way that particles, though made of the same components, do, and all prostheses, bulky as they are, behave in a still different way.

Now, let us consider two toxicological parameters: LD_{50} and LC_{50}.

LD_{50} (lethal dose fifty) is defined as the amount of a material, administered all at once, which kills 50% of a group of test animals. LD_{50} measures acute toxicity, that is, the short-term poisoning potential, of a certain material.

'LC_{50}' stands for 'lethal concentration fifty' and refers not to the quantity but to the concentration of a substance in air or in water which causes the death of half the animals used for the test [2].

The actual LD_{50} value may be, and often is, different for a certain substance, depending on the route of exposure (e.g. ingestion, transdermal, inhalation, etc.). These different values are obtained testing the chemicals on laboratory animals. Special calculations are used when translating animal LD_{50} values to possible lethal dose values for humans. Safety factors of 10,000 or 1000 are usually included in such calculations to allow for the variability between individuals and how they react to a chemical, and for the uncertainties of experiment test results.

The limits of the two parameters are self-evident. Among others, a given substance can be toxic for a certain tissue or organ without affecting others. An organ can be affected by a substance without it causing death. Another problem hard to solve is the comparison between different kinds of damage: How can one determine objectively whether a damage is more or less serious than another? What with a substance which is objectively noxious but does not cause death? How can one scientifically cope with the obvious difference existing among different test animals, and how can one scientifically translate the results to humans without being ready to accept a huge margin of error? Answers are not lacking, but understandably, none of them is totally reliable.

As far as substances is concerned, the key point is that particles, particularly nano ones, can enter freely into cells, and interact chemically – that is, through the substances in question – with other biological substances impairing or destroying the local metabolism. From a purely theoretical point of view, it is sufficient that a single cell is attacked and that, as will be seen later, its defenses are made unable to function, to trigger a very serious biological reaction.

For that reason, it was necessary to study ad hoc tests identifying suitable parameters.

Then, another definition of biocompatibility (1991) came to consider biomaterial as 'a material intended to interface with biological system to evaluate, treat, augment or replace any tissue, organ or function of the body'. It is only obvious that this implies that there is a tolerance on the part of the organism in respect of that material and tolerance must be evaluated by appropriate tests considering the actual acute, long-term and chronic effects of this interaction.

First of all, it is necessary to remember that the body invariably reacts to the entrance of something which does not belong there and is not recognised as self, with something which can vary from a complete rejection to a mild reaction to a temporary acceptance to, in the best of circumstances, full acceptance.

If a more or less quick rejection and a mild reaction are easy to understand, temporary acceptability needs some explanation. Biocompatibility may not be an eternal property of a certain material. In fact, a material, once implanted, can induce a slow, low-degree biological reaction, which, as a final result, can lead to discomfort, mild pathologies or even full rejection.

The material used to replace a function of the body (orthopaedic prostheses, cardiac valves, etc.) or a tissue (skin, tooth, bone, blood) inside the body is subjected to stress and to chemical and biological interactions with what is present in the body. It works, it ages and it can wear. A well-known case is that of hip joint prostheses losing surface debris due to the friction between counterparts. In this occurrence, the debris invades the neighbouring tissues and, as a rule, induces a biological reaction. Figure 2.1 presents schemes and X-ray images of hip joint prostheses.

The bulk material may have passed all tests and be declared biocompatible, but that is not the case with its debris. As a matter of fact, they are generally attacked by macrophages and moved to other parts of the body. Generally speaking, and with some exceptions, biological materials (bone, cells, etc.) can reconstruct themselves, but synthetic materials are always unable to do so. What they do is degrade, or due to the surface interaction with body fluids, they can change some of their properties as happens, for example, in the case of corrosion, an oxidation process which occurs also inside the body at 37°C in an aqueous environment full of chemicals and crossed by weak electric currents. As a rule, degradation and oxidation products are not compatible, and a relatively frequent example of that incompatibility is represented by the release of iron hydroxide, a quite common event when iron-based matter is for any reason inserted into the body. Besides having grown incompatible, the prosthesis becomes so more and more useless. In some circumstances, a prosthesis may remain relatively biocompatible but stops functioning as it should. This is the case, for example, of the formation of *bacterial biofilms* or a so-called *pannus* on heart valve prostheses, that is, an ingrowth of tissue.

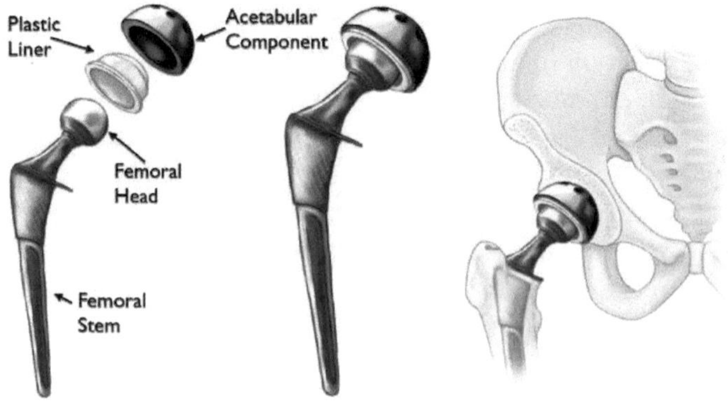

(a)

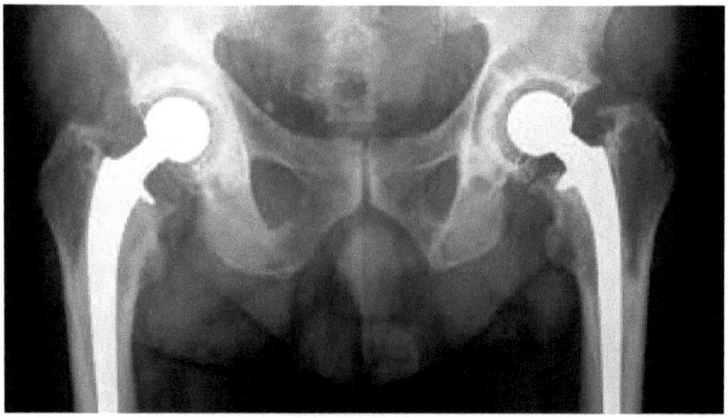

(b)

Figure 2.1 (a) Images show examples of hip joint prostheses made of metallic, ceramic and polymeric materials and (b) Rx images of different types of hip joint prostheses. Reproduced with permission from OrthoInfo © American Academy of Orthopaedic Surgeons (http://orthoino.aaos.org).

This behaviour suggested the opportunity of developing temporary implants (when it was the case) like those used, for instance, in case of bone fracture when helping the edges of the fracture to be in touch with each other is necessary in order to facilitate healing (intramedullary nail, osteosynthesis plate and nail, etc.). When the fracture is recovered, those devices are no longer necessary, so they can be removed. Of course, no temporary implants can be used in the case of physical impossibility by the body to heal or reconstruct itself.

On the other side, biodegradability can be a very useful property. In fact, surgical sutures are the oldest example, so that, once they have done their job, removal is no longer needed as they 'disappear'. It is the case of the so-called *catgut suture* (although cats have nothing to do with it). Connective tissue is taken from the small intestine of sheep, cattle, horses or pigs, after having undergone a chemical treatment, and now synthetic materials are used for internal sutures which have the peculiarity to be absorbed in a time longer than that it takes to the wound to heal.

As a matter of fact, non-degradable prostheses can wear during their use, and after a certain time they must be replaced in order to maintain their function. It is the case of hip joint prostheses which can wear and release wear debris which cause an inflammatory body reaction. In conclusion, bulk material can be biocompatible, but not its debris, and generally speaking, metal debris are more dangerous than ceramic or plastic ones.

An example of such a reaction is that caused by the metal–metal hip joint prosthesis called McKee–Farrar and a similar one produced, decades after, by DePuy (J&J) (Fig. 2.2a,b).

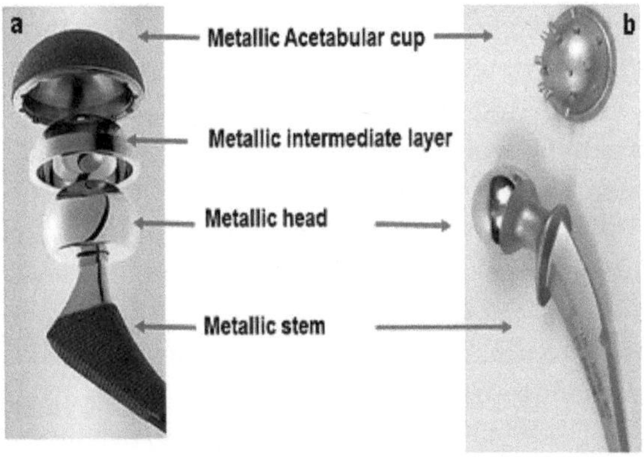

Figure 2.2 Images of two metal–metal hip joint prostheses: (a) the more recent one by DePuy and (b) the old McKee–Farrar one.

The studies on biomaterials and biocompatibility led to new concepts like that of the 'sandwich materials'. Since it is hardly possible to make an artificial material with all the properties requested (according to each case, strength, non-wettability, elasticity, softness, durability, etc.), researchers devised materials made of different layers, with every layer corresponding to a specific property. The new materials have a mechanically resistant core and their surface is coated with molecules as similar as possible to the biological matrix they have to match (*biomimetic coating*). There are also coatings which can be bioactive, meaning that they change over time (biodegradation process) in order to generate an *osteointegration*, that is, a direct bonding with the bone. That is the case of *bioglasses* [3, 4].

The concept is that the prosthesis is coated with something which 'cheats' the biological host which recognises it as self, and in some products the molecules are 'powered' in order to determine an intimate, close contact with the biological tissue. In some cases, that technology succeeds in developing structures (scaffolds) which can host cells of the patient. As far as material is concerned, these organic-inorganic devices are fully biocompatible, since they contain part of the hosting body, and that part is in touch with the subject's tissues. The outlook seems to be in the hands of tissue engineering and synthetic biology [5].

A branch of implantology is related to tissue engineering. That involves the new concept of *self-regeneration*. In some particular cases of implantology, it is possible to stress the self-regeneration of a tissue or function. The scientist prepares a scaffold (a resistant armature) which is seeded (filled) with the previously explanted cells of the patient, which are cultivated and expanded. To maximise the expansion, growth factors can be added to the culture broth. In this case, the patient will receive something which is particularly biocompatible. For example, an ear has been reconstructed for aesthetic reasons (Fig. 2.3).

A big boost to prosthesis production comes from 3D technology. Born to reproduce small things such as toys, 3D printing is increasingly proving to be an exceptional tool to produce customised prostheses as well as in various specialties of surgery [6]. This new method allows us to manufacture prostheses built exactly on the patient, with obviously better results than those obtained from industrial products, which can also be of the highest quality but, however, mass-produced without being able to take into account the individual case.

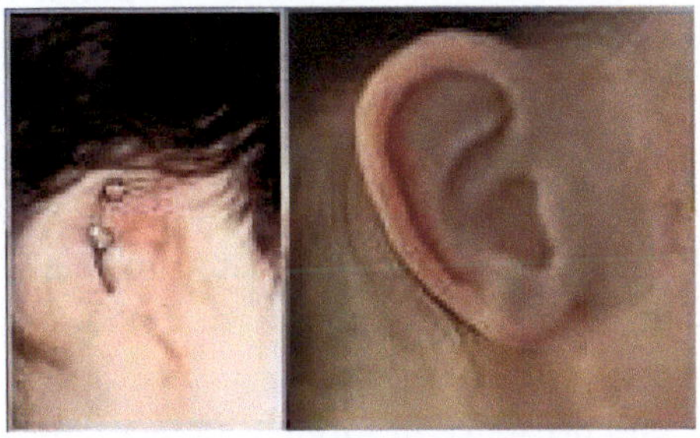

Figure 2.3 Ear prosthesis. Image of a head without one ear (left) and 3D reconstruction with a polymeric prosthesis made on a copy of the other ear (right). Figure courtesy of Professor L. Di Silvio.

2.2 Particles in the Tissues

As occurs in all circumstances with foreign bodies, *macrophages*, the phagocytic cells of the innate immune system, are quickly attracted to the spot, their main function being that of engulfing foreign agents which, for any reason and no matter how, had managed to enter the body. This includes particulate matter. Macrophages have also the capacity to secrete in a very short time a wide range of inflammatory mediators, among which *cytokines*, small proteins influencing the development and extent of the inflammatory response. Inflammation, a mechanism of innate immunity, serves to eliminate the initial cause of cell injury, clear out necrotic cells and tissues damaged from the insult they underwent and start the process of tissue repair. If the inflammatory reaction is not big enough, the condition could lead to progressive tissue destruction by the original damaging agent (e.g. bacteria) and put at risk the very survival of the whole organism. Chronic inflammation is characterised by the presence of mononuclear cells, mainly macrophages, and by phenomena of simultaneous destruction and healing of the tissue involved, a combination which can lead to a host of pathologies, including cancer. Inflammation by particles is both relatively mild and, if particles are not degradable, chronic, thus representing an impending danger to the organism.

Once the foreign bodies have been engulfed by macrophages, their function is that of digesting them: apoptotic cells, microbes and other organic foreign bodies. But solid, inorganic, insoluble particles are not digestible. So, when those particles are involved, macrophages, though actually engulfing them, are useless and can only do as much as secreting substances inducing inflammation.

Particularly when a fair number of particles are grouped in a limited volume, an inflammatory, granulation tissue grows, wrapping and isolating them from the surrounding cells.

In all cases, the presence of foreign bodies induces a biological reaction of the tissues. The consequent inflammation can achieve various effects: from becoming a cancer, normally a slow process, to modifying the patient's behaviour when it affects the brain or, as it looks more and more likely, modifying the intestinal microbiota, through a range of other pathological effects.

In the texts of laws and regulations in force worldwide, particles are often mentioned, when they are mentioned at all, as 'inert'. Incinerator bottom ash is an example. If the classification, even though far from irrefutably correct, may be accepted from a chemical standpoint, it is thoroughly wrong if biological activity, that is, what is really important from people's health's point of view, is considered. In most cases, the particles we deal with are crystals or amorphous structures with a poor or a completely not appreciable chemical reactivity, but in all cases, they are foreign bodies with an enormous biological reactivity, initially as inflammation inducers, and lawmakers and their advisers should take this into due account.

2.3 Biocompatibility and Nanotechnologies

As can be seen, nowadays the concept of biocompatibility has changed dramatically.

But now we have a new challenge to face: the biocompatibility of nanoparticles and *nanobiosafety*, that is, the degree of safety of particles when they enter the body, always taking into account the enormous variety in which particles exist.

Through nanotechnologies, a lot of objects with unique, often surprising, characteristics are being produced and they are introduced also in medicine, with a view to solve old problems by using novel materials or nanotechnological devices.

Nanoparticles are called 'magic bullets' for their ability to cross any physiological barriers. In single form or in clusters, nanoparticles can enter cells and interact with organelles, proteins and enzymes at the nanolevel. For reasons which have to do both with science and the 'bureaucratic' convenience of placing numbers as limits, to be nano, a particle, be it crystalline or amorphous, must not exceed a 0.1 μm size. Particles that size have very peculiar properties which become more and more evident as the ratio between external surface and volume increases or, which is the same thing, as their size grows smaller. So, particles like those are more and more often produced in laboratories with steric properties and chemical compositions studied depending on the use to which they are intended. In fact, they are used in growing applications which can be found in nanotechnology textbooks, constantly trying to keep up with the continuous, faster and faster innovations and applications of engineered nanoparticles.

Nanobiointeraction is the key point to be checked to assess the biocompatibility of nanoparticles. That implies their behaviour when in touch with cells, proteins, enzymes, etc. The evaluation of the relationships between cellular uptake and a toxic response (Trojan horse effect) is a new frontier, difficult to deal with both for the limited knowledge we have of it and for the difficulties of investigations we face. We do not know well enough what processes determine the toxic potential necessary, for instance, to a pro-oxidant activity. We do not know that there is the possibility for the cell to excrete those nanosized foreign bodies and get rid of them the way it happens with non-biocompatible implants or devices [7].

What will matter for what we are dealing with in this chapter is that particles that size, be they engineered or, much more commonly, the product of unintentional pollution, have a toxicity which, as already pointed out, is quite different from that shown by bulkier material with the same chemistry.

Their most evident feature is their capability of crossing virtually any physiological barrier without being perceived, and it is for that reason that they are called not only magic but also 'invisible bullets'. They are so good at penetrating everywhere that they can enter cell nuclei and interfere with proteins, with chemicals like, for instance, enzymes, with organelles and even with the DNA. This cross-relationship (nanobiointeraction [8]) is crucial in assessing biocompatibility, and chemistry is but one of the parameters to be considered, not the most important, size and shape being more determining though not the sole.

With nanoparticles, dose keeps being important à la Paracelsus, but other parameters need be considered. As a matter of fact, we don't know what the exact circumstances are to allow particles to enter cell nuclei, nor do we know why very often they stay outside cells, but, again as a matter of fact, when particles cross a cell membrane they can cause dramatic consequences, and dose becomes just a minor actor, being that only a parameter which can increase or decrease the degree of likelihood which makes the phenomenon occur. In short, in this case, Paracelsus's concept of dose becomes a variation of probability. Anyhow, at least from a theoretical point of view, a single cell into which a particle has penetrated and has interfered with the DNA can be the trigger for an extremely important pathological reaction. It should be kept in mind that the DNA attacked in that way loses the ability to repair itself and the cell loses its apoptosis capacity. So that the daughter cell is the result of modified genetic information and reproduction with the inherited, modified DNA will continue as long as the tissue receives its nourishment.

Again, as size is concerned, the smaller it is and, as a consequence, the higher is the outer surface/volume ratio, the more energy is contained in the particle (a feature which nanotechnologists widely exploit). That energy exerts an influence on the surrounding cells, an influence which needs to be explored in detail and which is far or, in any case, different from the old dose concept.

Another parameter which has nothing to do with dose is the shape particles have. For merely mechanical reasons, spherical particles like those generated at high temperature, for example, when melting metals, are less capable of moving across tissues than many irregularly shaped particles or needle-shaped ones. And size and shape combined together are also critical. In addition to being richer in energy due to the large surface/volume ratio, a particle with a particularly jagged surface offers a large contact to tissues and that must necessarily have a significance.

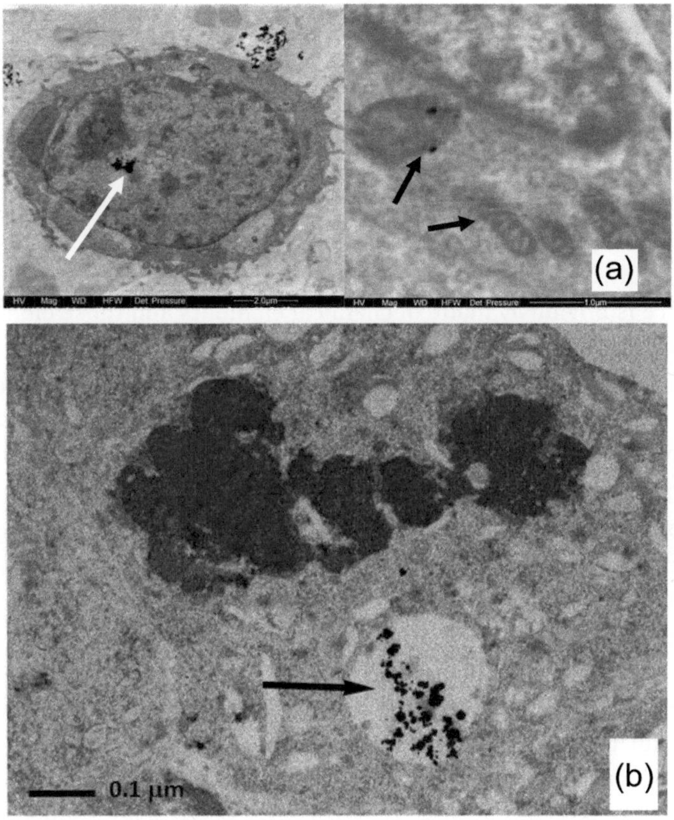

Figure 2.4 (a) In vitro tests of cells with iron oxide nanoparticles. A fibroblastic cell is shown in contact with iron oxide nanoparticles (white arrow). Some nanoparticles remain outside the cell, but others can enter and interact with mitochondria (black arrows), inducing alteration and the ensuing damage in the cell metabolism. They do not induce cell death, and the cell can go into mitosis. When the nuclear membrane disappears, the particles (black arrow) are very likely to interact with DNA (see panel b), which acquires erroneous information, becoming unable to remedy it and becoming unable to die from apoptosis. (b) Iron oxide nanoparticles (black arrow) close to chromatin (DNA).

Incidentally, it must also be remembered that some particles, especially those produced by high-temperature processes like those typical of foundries and incinerators, are often hollow inside with a very fragile surface. That surface gets easily crumbled into very tiny fragments, besides having an increased number of particles following the breakup.

But particles can also be electrically charged, and that is obviously important when they get in touch with tissues or with chemicals like, for example, proteins. In the latter case, proteins can be altered either chemically or sterically by unfolding processes, thus changing their characteristics. Just as a theme suggested to researchers for further studies, enzymes have a protein nature and altering them can be a cause of consequences hard to predict.

Finally, chemistry has an influence on how particles behave. Their surface is obviously made of chemical elements and those elements keep, at least in part, their toxicity, if any. But even here, not all is so simple. We may take steel here as an easy example. Steel, an alloy of iron atoms with varying amounts of carbon and other elements, is usually a crystal with an internal structure made up of neat rows of atoms. In addition to iron, which is the main component, and carbon, the most common elements present in steel are generally chromium and nickel. When a stainless-steel implant is inserted in the body, the reactions which tissues show to it are not those they would deploy against iron, chromium or nickel alone. The same thing occurs with particles.

As can be easily deduced, it is impossible to establish simple rules for the behaviour of particles, these being very different from each other for a set of dimensional, steric, electrical, radiological and chemical characteristics. So, the toxicology of particles is much more complex than Paracelsus's one, simplistically applying which is an endless source of misunderstanding and blunders.

Only when doctors have acquired these fundamental notions in their cultural background, the more and more numerous health problems caused by the particles which we keep introducing into our lives will get a hope to be remedied.

2.4 How Particles Behave in the Body

We have already described in detail in our book *Nanopathology: The Health Impact of Nanoparticles* (Pan Stanford Publishing, 2008, now Jenny Stanford Publishing) how solid, inorganic micro- and nanoparticles which are insoluble in water and fats are generated.

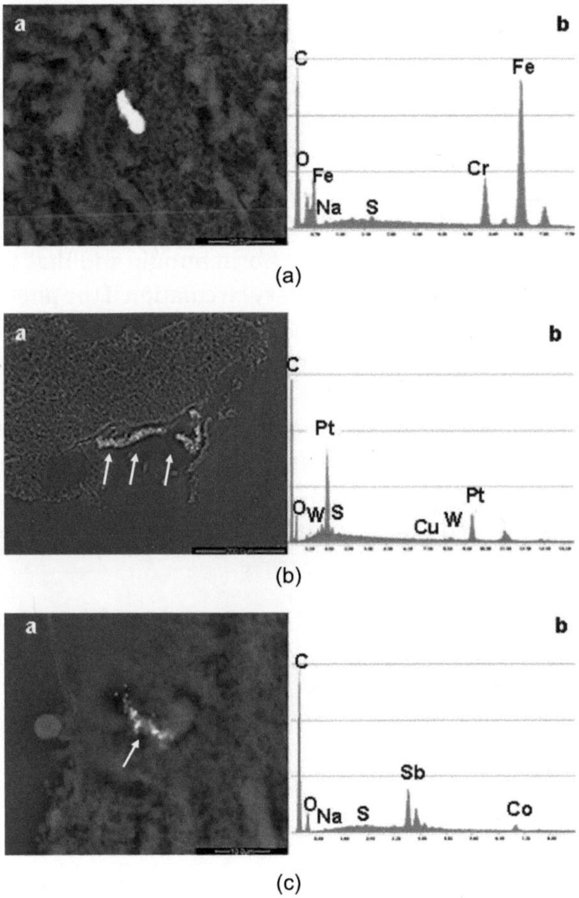

Figure 2.5 Micro- and nanosized foreign bodies detected inside a thrombus entrapped in a vena cava filter explanted from a patient who suffered from clotting disorders. In the three cases shown by electron microscopy images, it is clear how the particles which entered the blood, however they entered it, transformed the fibrinogen into fibrin, thereby constituting the scaffold for a thrombus. The elemental chemical analyses of the particles show different compositions (compounds of Fe-Cr-Ni, Pt, Sb-Co,) which have led to the same result, thereby demonstrating once again that by far the most relevant factor triggering the reaction is being a foreign body, regardless of other characteristics of the particles.

Next we will concisely summarise the basic concepts.

Their mass can be even millions of times smaller than that of a pollen, and therefore, particles float easily in the atmosphere, behaving in several ways as if they were a gas. For this reason, they are inhaled and breathed, being able to end up in the pulmonary alveoli, where they remain generally a few tens of seconds, negotiate the alveolar barrier and enter the bloodstream. Here, in a minority of subjects, those who do not have an efficient fibrinolytic system, the particles transform the soluble protein fibrinogen present in the plasma into the insoluble protein fibrin.

Then, a thrombus forms on the fibrin bundle and that thrombus necessarily migrates to the pulmonary circulation if the phenomenon has occurred within the veins. The consequence is a pulmonary thrombo-embolism, a condition in which, depending on the vascular trunks which are occluded, one or more areas of the lungs are excluded and, if the area is large enough, death can be the result.

In the event that the phenomenon occurs within the arteries, the embolising thrombus can end up in any body district, preventing the arrival of oxygenated blood to that particular tissue – hence, events such as myocardial infarction or stroke.

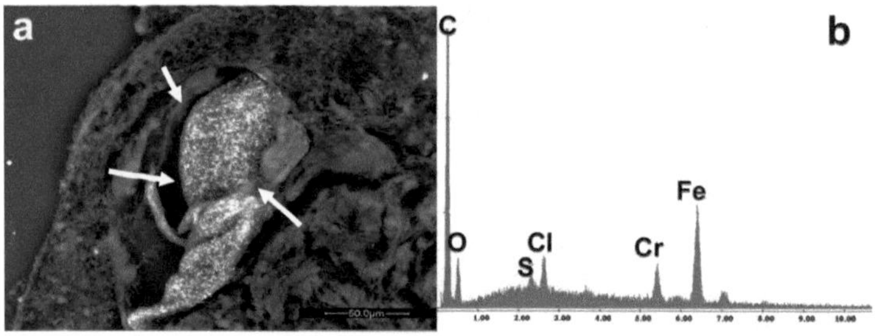

Figure 2.6 Thrombus extracted from an infarcted coronary vessel. The electron microscopy images show three cases of thrombi removed by means of a thrombolyser from heart attack patients. All the thrombi contained foreign bodies surrounded by blood components. In this case there is a cluster of steel nanoparticles (white arrows). Their biointeraction triggered the transformation of fibrinogen into fibrin, thereby making up the scaffold for a thrombus.

In the majority of subjects, though, if a thrombus has formed, it is immediately dissolved[a] and the particles travel carried by the

[a]Fibrinolysis, the process of breaking down and dissolving a thrombus, is very quick in happening, mainly due to plasmin, the serine protease that, among other important functions, can degrade many blood plasma proteins, including fibrin clots.

blood, virtually able to reach any organ or tissue, with destinations impossible to predict. As soon as the particle reaches the end of its journey, the tissue where it has arrived behaves like any mechanical filter, capturing it.

It is at this stage that the particles can be attacked by macrophages which incorporate them and take them elsewhere where they go to die, leaving organic residues which the body easily eliminates. The particle, however, is not degradable and remains where it was moved by the macrophage.

The particles, be they where they ended after being moved by the macrophages or where the blood had brought them, according to a well-known mechanism of reaction to foreign bodies, are wrapped in a tissue (granulation tissue) which remains chronically inflamed and which, in times which can be very long, gives rise to cancer. In many circumstances, the time required for cancer to become clinically manifest is longer than the life of the individual and, therefore, the process goes unnoticed. To avoid misunderstandings, it is necessary to clarify that the type of cancer which is thus generated depends on many different factors, including the organ affected, its health, the quantity of particles involved, their shape, their size, their chemical constitution, their physical characteristics, the presence of any contributing causes, etc.

As already mentioned, particles can penetrate inside the cells up to the nucleus, where they interfere in an unpredictable way with the DNA and take away from the cell the ability to repair itself and to resort to apoptosis as a last possibility of defense of the common good of all the cells of the organ involved and, ultimately, of the whole organism. Thus, the cell with the modified DNA reproduces, following incorrect instructions and, deprived of its ability to apoptosis, continues to reproduce erroneously as long as it is nourished.

This event is that which makes the main difference between classical toxicology and nanotoxicology and it is the key to understanding many diseases of unknown origin, like cancer.

But particles can also cause diseases which have nothing to do with cancer.

Among these, is type 1 diabetes, in which particles, by reaching the pancreas, prevent beta cells of the islets of Langerhans from producing insulin. Reaching the brain, they can trigger behavioural pathologies (e.g. aggressiveness, perhaps autism, Parkinson's disease, Alzheimer's disease, etc.). Going from the mother to the foetus without difficulty, they can cause abortions or malformations or induce cancer in the foetus.

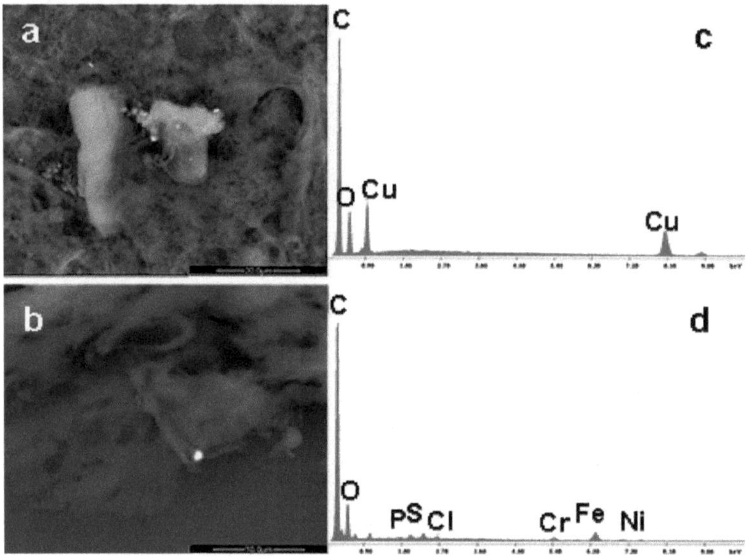

Figure 2.7 Case of a baby with cancer of the yolk sac. The images show the findings of particles within the yolk sac cancer in an infant. Particles of stainless steel (iron-chromium-nickel) have been detected, very common among urban polluting dust, and, together with those, copper-based particles of which we could not identify the origin. To do so, it would have been necessary to investigate at least the environment in which the mother (in an excellent health condition) lived, her activity, her diet and any medications she was taking.

As is evident, micro- and nanoparticles can cause seemingly very different diseases. About 20 years ago, we grouped all those diseases by calling them *nanopathologies*, a name which, with its prefix 'nano', could lead to the error that these are diseases of little relevance. In fact, they are not only often very serious but also widespread. Not a few of them are still considered cryptogenic, that is, of unknown origin or of uncertain origin.

The willingness to accept or, at least, to consider without obtusely refusing a priori possibilities other than the traditional ones could facilitate progress, leading to a better diagnostic capacity, more effective therapies and prevention strategies which avoid contracting the disease, that is, primary prevention, which, of all strategies, is the most effective and by far the least expensive.

2.5 Objections to Particle Theory

One of the most common objections to particle theory – as long as it's actually a theory and not something objective observable by anyone who really wants to do it – is, 'If dust is everywhere and is actually pathogenic, we should all get sick.' The objection is the same as the one advanced more than a century and a half ago against Pasteur: 'If microbes are everywhere and they are actually pathogenic, we should all get sick.' *Polymorphism* is the main answer biology gives now to counter the objection as to microbes, that is, a phenomenon of differentiation of some DNA genes which, not for all people but for some of them, adapt by natural selection: a phenomenon subject to certain conditions, including the meeting between pathogens and the body, granting it the capacity to react defensively against the pathogens with the possibility of causing the disease. Then, account must be taken of how the body has a number of defense mechanisms grouped in its *immune system*. Those conditions may somehow apply to particles as well, but as much as we know now, there is no evidence.

But the answer must also concern many other aspects of exposure to particles.

Just to give some examples, nobody undergoes exactly the same exposure in terms of quantity, quality and exposure times. Admitting to having a group of never-exposed subjects and to letting them breathe the same quantity and quality of particles, each of them, according to the capabilities of their respiratory system, will exhale different quantities, and on the other hand, each of them will block different amounts in the lung alveoli. For example, smokers, with their underactive, when not altogether paralysed, vibritile cilia, and with the layer of mucus coating their airways, will be less able to get rid of the particles.

In practical terms, such a simple situation as the one just hypothesised is in fact impossible, given that each of us has a different history of exposure, of course, not only to particles but to a huge number of poisons, and as is a well-known notion in toxicology, when numerous different toxic substances act simultaneously, the result is unpredictable and, in any case, is more serious than the arithmetic sum of the single effects.

Another parameter to consider is the state of health of the subject and, in particular, of the target organ of the particles. In particular, a hyperemic organ because it is inflamed, just because it receives an excess of blood, has an increased chance of receiving particulate matter. Again by way of example, the particles can reach the brain by crossing the blood–brain barrier when, together with them, particular substances are present. These include, for example, glyphosate, a non-selective herbicide which pollutes many vegetable food products, and polysorbate80, an emulsifier currently used in vaccines: a type of combined exposure which takes place only occasionally.

Ultimately, due to the great difference which exists between individuals and even in the same individual during his/her life up to variations which occur during the day, it is at least naive as well as being in contrast with the objectivity of science to expect that every man behaves exactly like his neighbour. Such a thing is possible with a very small margin of error only in unicellular beings. When reproduction is sexual with the meeting of different DNAs, as organisms grow more complex, the differences between individuals become more and more marked until they reach the maximum in *Homo sapiens*. This top of complexity exists not because we are biologically more complex than any primate but because, among other peculiarities, we have a psyche capable of interfering (chemically) with our physiology much more than it does in any other animal.

Though we are aware of that, our current knowledge does not allow us to establish to what extent this peculiarity can affect micro- and nanoparticulate diseases.

References

1. Williams, D. (2008). Biocompatibility. *Tissue Engineering*, Academic Press, pp. 255–278, https://doi.org/10.1016/B978-0-12-370869-4.00009-4.
2. https://ccohs.ca/oshanswers/chemicals/ld50.html.

3. Gatti, A. and Monari, E. (1998). Bioactivity of the active glasses. *New Biomedical Materials: Basic and Applied Studies*, Haris, P. I. and Chapman D., eds., IOS Press Amsterdam, pp. 73–80, ISBN 90 5199 365.
4. Gatti, A., Hench, L., Monari, E., Gonella, I., and Caccavale, M. (1997). Test of Bioactivity in four different glasses. *Bioceramics*, Vol. 10, Sedel, L. and Rey, C., eds., Elsevier Science Ltd., Paris, pp. 287–290.
5. https://en.wikipedia.org/wiki/Synthetic_biology.
6. https://www.burtonnitta.co.uk/NewOrgansOfCreation.html.
7. http://www.drug-dev.com/Main/Back-Issues/NANOTECHNOLOGY-MARKET-Nanotechnology-Markets-in-He-803.aspx.
8. Gatti, A. (2016). Nano-biointeraction and nanopathology. *News Medical Life Sciences*, http://www.news-medical.net/news/20161031/Nano-biointeraction-andnanopathology.aspx.

Chapter 3

How Nanoparticles Are Generated

3.1 What Are Particles and How Are They Produced?

As already mentioned, a few natural sources of particles are present on our planet. Volcanic eruptions are the most dramatic and showy among them. To be sure, unlike what happened a few tens of millions of years ago, not many volcanoes are active nowadays, but when occasionally they belch out, the environmental consequences, though generally short-lived, are often very visible. The year 1816 was known as the 'year without summer' because of the severe climate abnormalities caused by the eruption of the Dutch East Indies Mount Tambora, which reached its climax in April 1815 and continued to emit fumes and particulate matter for about three more years. Its dust occupied a large portion of the atmosphere in the northern hemisphere, thus preventing the sun rays and heat to reach the lower atmosphere and the ground in the usual and, for us, necessary way and causing, among other problems, the scarcity or the utter lack of crops. About two centuries later, in 2010, the Icelandic Eyjafjallajökull erupted and its dust forced some European airports to close for a few days. About 1500 are the still potentially active volcanoes, more or less one-third of which, mainly located in the so-called Pacific Ring, have erupted in historical time. In any

Advances in Nanopathology: From Vaccines to Food
Antonietta Morena Gatti and Stefano Montanari

ISBN 978-981-4877-29-9 (Hardcover), 978-1-003-05622-5 (eBook)
www.jennystanford.com

case, apart from rather rare exceptions, volcanic dust is not a great danger to health and the environment.

Rock erosion due to ageing and climate (wind, rain, ice, etc.) or, more seldom, landslides are another source of particulate matter. Those particles are generally bigger than volcanoes and, because of that, are not particularly aggressive, since, if inhaled, they are blocked in the upper respiratory tract or, if ingested, they are often too coarse to cross the wall of the digestive system (though those walls are rather permeable) and are eliminated with faeces.

In spite of their size, large enough to be easily visible, sand grains mostly raised by the wind from desert areas can travel over very long distances. Sahara sand, for example, reaches the East Coast of America and can be found in the red rain which occasionally falls in Europe. The Mongolian Gobi Desert's sand is often carried by the wind to Beijing and other Chinese cities.

Forest fires, very rarely natural in their cause and much more often set by arsonists or reckless goers, are a further source of dust. As we are writing these pages (early 2020), the hugest forest fire in the history of man is taking place in southeast Australia, with the particles produced by combustion which have already reached South America, covering no less than 12,000 km, and for a comparatively long time the situation appeared to be out of control. Millions of hectares of land were involved, and both the heat and the disappearance of vegetation prevented the formation of cloud bodies and, therefore, the fall of rain. What is happening is the outbreak of lightning without thunderstorms which triggers new fire outbreaks.

In most circumstances, it is man who is responsible for the formation of particularly polluting dust, and that is a rocketing increase whose entire consequences can only be a matter of speculation, since there is no experience in that matter, except for acute cases. One of them, for example, was the so-called Great Smog which affected London from Friday, 5 December, to Tuesday, 9 December 1952. Particularly cold weather combined with atmospheric high pressure and windless conditions collected airborne pollutants mostly due to the use of coal as a fuel for home heating. That combination of pollutants formed a thick layer of smog over the city, which, according to recent evaluations, caused about 12,000 fatalities.

As happened then in London, most man-produced particles originate from combustion. Temperature is usually high enough to break the molecules of what is being burned, reducing them to smaller molecules or to atoms. If the formation of particles from those fragments of matter is completed immediately in the neighbourhood where the combustion occurs, those particles are called *filterable*, because, if a filter is placed downstream of the phenomenon, it can ideally capture them. When, instead, the formation occurs at a farther distance from combustion, small molecules and atoms pass freely through the filter and stick together. In that case the particles are *condensable*. In both eventualities, the elementary composition of the resulting particles is different from that of each of the original substances which have been burned. The atomic elements are obviously the same, but their combination is random, more or less as if we had a mosaic, we disassembled it and then recombined its tiles with eyes closed. It should be noted that the formation of particles also takes place by burning material which is not solid but liquid, such as, for example, automotive or power plant fuel, or gaseous, such as, for example, that generated by the combustion of industrial methane.

The third category of particulate matter created at high temperature is the *secondary*. Combustion releases different gases, depending on the composition of what is being burned: particularly carbon oxides, sulphur dioxide, nitrogen oxides, ammonia and a quantity of different volatile organic compounds. Once in the atmosphere, they find oxygen, also as its allotropic form ozone, free radicals, water vapour and a mixture of gases varying from place to place, from situation to situation and from time to time, occasionally changing in a matter of hours. In a time which in some instances takes days, catalysed by the sun and, more in particular, by the ultraviolet rays, a condensation reaction takes place among all those gases, forming new particles, precisely the secondary ones. Besides being definitely more numerous than filterable and condensable primary particles, the secondary ones have an important feature: organic pollutants, like, for instance, dioxins and furans, stick to them and are carried by them even to relatively long distances. Due to the time which condensation takes and because of diffusion phenomena, secondary particles can be found pretty far from the actual source of the substances by which they have been generated, and the pollutants adhering to them can have origins which have little or nothing to do with that of the particles themselves.

Though, at least hopefully, not a usual form of dust pollution typical of man, the collapse of the Twin Towers in New York on 11 September 2001, is a particularly important one, immediately followed as it was by a huge cloud of dust, much of which had a particularly fine size because of the very high temperature reached. According to some information sources, apart from the many thousands of tons of concrete, the rest consisted of more than 2500 contaminants: roughly 50% non-fibrous material and construction debris, 40% glass and other fibres, 9.2% cellulose and 0.8% of asbestos, plus lead and mercury, not to mention the variety of metals contained in computers and other electronic systems. That dust lingered for a long time in the atmosphere before, eventually, falling to the ground, probably also far away from the place where the cloud started. It is reasonable to assume that some of the dust has entered into many air-conditioning pipelines with all its obvious consequences.

A much more usual man-made high-temperature production is that coming from explosions.

Of this, as of 9/11, more will be said later.

Not all man-produced particles come from high-temperature processes. If not equally important in terms of quantity, friction can produce dust as well. Turning works in factories and workshops and the brake pads of cars rubbing against discs, for example, are dust producers.

The particles we deal with and which are discussed in this book are solid and inorganic. Their size varies from a few tens of nanometres up to a few tens of microns. By official definition, nanoparticles (or ultrafine particles) have a size ranging from 1 to 100 nm. Again officially, fine particles are sized between 100 nm and 2.5 μm, while coarse particles cover a range between 2.5 and 10 μm. In our research field, that classification has no great meaning. So, in general, we call nanoparticles those whose size is smaller than 1 μm and microparticles the ones larger than that size. It is just a matter of personal habit and of convenience, which, of course, is of no consequence, though deemed important by those who approach science in a bureaucratic way.

If particles vary greatly in size, their shape is at least as variable. A sphere or a spheroid is often the result of high-temperature processes, particularly when metals like, for example, iron are involved. In a way, those shapes remind one of soap bubbles: a formation which is hollow inside and is surrounded by an outer, thin, solid crust. That crust, the outer surface of the sphere, is generally composed of juxtaposed crystals, which make the structure very fragile, and because of that, it crumbles easily, thus producing 'shards' whose size is obviously much smaller than the original particle and whose shape looks geometrically irregular.

If temperature is not high enough to produce spheres, the shapes of the particles can't be guessed.

As already briefly mentioned, size is roughly inversely proportional to the temperature of formation: the higher the temperature, the smaller the particle.

It must be kept in mind that, because it is extremely important and will be useful later, for their evaluation as environmental pollutants, particles are considered as if they were spheres and, therefore, have a radius. It is also to be recalled that the volume of a sphere is proportional to the third power of the radius (the volume of a sphere is calculated multiplying 4/3 by π by the radius cubed). Therefore, if a sphere has a radius 10 times greater than that of another sphere, its volume is 10^3, that is, 1000, times greater.

When the origin of a particle happens to be a friction, that particle has often, though not in all cases, sharp edges.

All these notions, along with the chemical composition of the particulate matter, are essential when one has to look for the origin of a particular pollution.

Very often, the inorganic particles produced by pollution are not easily degradable either in the environment and the biological tissues. So, they resist virtually unchanged for very long periods of time, in many circumstances far exceeding any human lifespan. This fact entails important problems, for example, their accumulation. Even if one tries to reduce pollution, in our case the introduction of particles, in the environment or in the body, their numbers and their density are inevitably destined to increase. Corrosion phenomena converting metals to a more stable form (e.g. oxide, hydroxide, sulphide) can transform particles into something else, occasionally no less toxic to the organism than the original.

The laboratory generation of nanoparticles, the so-called engineered nanoparticles (to be distinguished from incidental nanoparticles), is completely different. In that case, the particles are produced on purpose for industrial use and, therefore, have the desired shape and composition. Thus, when in a polluted sample all particles equal in shape and composition are found, one is almost certainly faced with engineered material. This concept is particularly important when, later in this book, we will talk about the pollutants of drugs, especially vaccines. In those cases, as far as we are concerned, we never found particles which could make one think of a purpose-made material, and everything we found appeared to be incidental pollution from inaccurate production methods and controls.

3.2 Waste: The Production of Incidental Nanoparticles

We have already pointed it out: man has characteristics which are unique among all creatures living on earth. Among them, we produce waste and we need energy. Of course, in spite of what most of us firmly believe, those are not primary needs nor are they a right, as man is an animal just like any primate and for at least 15,000 centuries has lived the way any ape does. And apes neither produce waste (at least not materials nature can't reuse) nor need energy (at least, not of the type employed by humans). But, though with enormous time differences among different places, more or less half a million years ago, man started to know how to light fire and, later, how to use it to make artifacts. It was then that man began to differentiate himself significantly, not in anatomy or physiology but in ethology, from any other animal, producing naturally unusable waste and using energy which was not naturally given.

Until relatively recently, waste was not a particular problem: the number and habits of the world's human population were easily compatible with the planet's 'physiology' or, better, they were tolerable, and for both technical and economic reasons, man did not produce large quantities of objects, nor did his technical procedures leave too much waste.

Nowadays, particularly in the course of the last century, each individual started to use and 'need' more and more objects, each of which required the use of materials and of energy to be manufactured, each of which had a shorter and shorter usable life (nowadays many products have a planned obsolescence), becoming inevitably true waste, that is, something which nature is at a loss with and does not know how to deal with. Nor, it must be admitted, is nature interested in doing, as the world always finds a balance, even if it is not certain that the new one will be something compatible with the prospering of human life.

Some decades ago, when plastics began to be widely used to make more and more numerous products, making them less expensive and, therefore, more within the reach of a growing number of people, the illusion was that we would spare natural resources, though plastics are made of oil, which is obviously a natural resource. The situation now, just after a very short time as compared with our presence in this planet, is that we have huge quantities of plastic waste we don't know how to cope with.

And, facing an ever-growing demand, energy and its supply too are becoming a problem. As a matter of fact and with few exceptions, however with little significance, the energy coming, be it directly or indirectly, from the sun is the only one living beings, humans, animals and vegetables alike, have available and have ever used. Though it is delivered in a quantity far exceeding our 'necessities', without getting into an argument which can't be part of this book, we are not technically able to use it, nor are we willing, except to a very small degree. So, we are forced to resort to sources coming not from without but from within the closed system which is the earth, by this condemning humanity to run out of supplies by a time which is still difficult to predict but which sooner or later will inevitably come. In short, if we use the fuel contained in a tank without the possibility of the tank being refilled, there is no escape: sooner or later the tank will be empty.

Regardless of how we get rid of waste in an uncontrolled manner, much of what we discard ends up in landfills: by no means a satisfactory solution. The technological way adopted in most cases to solve the more and more embarrassing problem, then, is that of burning waste with the advantageous side effect of obtaining precious energy.

But, as to energy, if calculations are done correctly and all data are duly taken into consideration without forgetting, underestimating or neglecting any of them, burning involves a loss-making budget, since the manufacture of what is burned requires quantities of energy which far exceed what is obtained by combustion. But, apart from this aspect whose discussion cannot belong in this book, one of the many demonstrations of how much man prefers to consider what is convenient for him at the moment by pretending that facts do not exist, account must be taken of the principle of conservation of mass according to which matter can't be destroyed but only transformed. So, scientifically speaking, waste is not eliminated but only transformed into something else.

Burning implies the oxidation, in fact the addition of atmospheric oxygen, of the substances which can be oxidised, and, for technical reasons, considering all the technology needed, combustion in an incinerator requires not only oxygen but also water, methane, activated carbon, carbonates, ammonia, etc. All this means adding to waste more or less as much mass, a mass which is then inevitably discharged as such or transformed into different pollutants into the environment. But, as already mentioned and leaving aside the thousands of organic pollutants (among which dioxins, furans, polychlorobiphenyls, a huge variety of polycyclic organic compounds, etc.), combustion means producing primary and secondary particles which, also as ash (approximately 1/3 of the initial waste mass is transformed into ash), enter the environment and accumulate. When treated legally, ash is disposed of in landfills and, being particularly toxic, makes this means of miscellaneous waste storage definitely dangerous. In some circumstances, we worked in landfills obtained from disused quarries, with the ashes which, together with a set of other toxic substances, carried by rainwater ended up in the aquifers. Mixed with asphalt, as it happens in some circumstances, that toxic ash constitutes a further risk to health, as asphalt gets rapidly worn, thus liberating those particles into the atmosphere. All in all, a similar risk is that of ashes mixed with cement, with the aggravating circumstance of obtaining a poor-quality product. More will be said in a few pages.

We have already described the formation of primary and secondary particles. Now, neglecting other details which are not part of this discussion, it should be remembered that air is a mixture composed of roughly one-fifth of oxygen and four-fifths of nitrogen. When this mixture is heated above a certain temperature, a temperature which is easily reached by waste incinerators and internal combustion engines, the two gases react together and give origin to nitrogen oxides (NOx): substances which are harmful both to the environment and to health.

No matter what technology is used, because of what (for us, modern humans) is an unfavourable natural law, not the least fraction of waste is eliminated, being it just transformed into something by far more toxic than the original. The 'advantage' is that combustion makes waste invisible to the eye, but unfortunately – and this is the con – very visible to the rest of our organism.

It is certainly a truism: the only acceptable waste with regard to the environment and health is that which is not produced.

When these obviousnesses are noticed, the most frequent reaction is to be told that whoever mentions them is an enemy of progress and would like to go back to the Stone Age. None of this: it is only a matter of realising how things are according to science.

We had a few chances to analyse ash from incinerators (Figs. 3.1–3.4) and fallen particles (Fig. 3.2) and other pollutants around some industries.

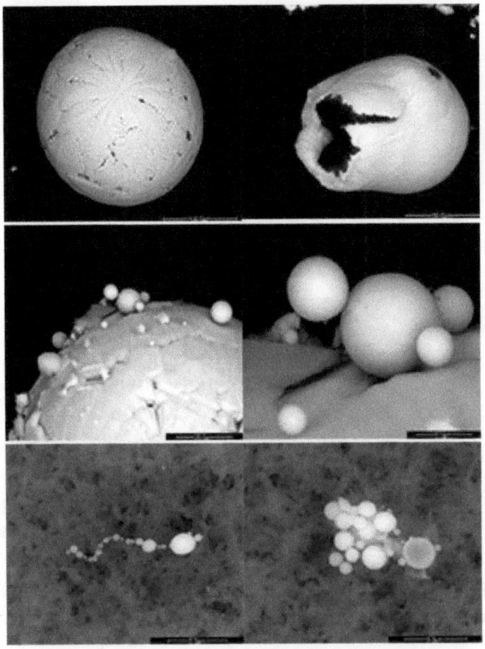

Figure 3.1 Spherical particles emitted by an incineration plant.

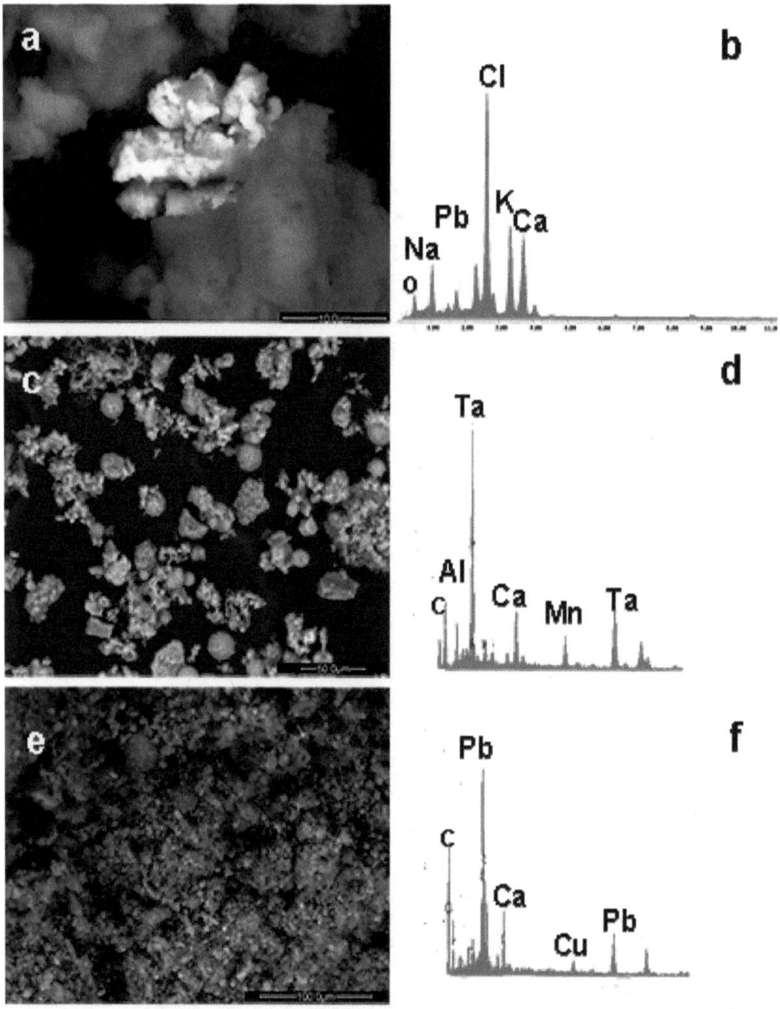

Figure 3.2 Ashes from an incinerator plant (Raibano, Italy). The ash shown in the images was collected in close vicinity of a waste incinerator plant placed in North Italy. As always when it comes to an origin from mixed waste, its composition is extremely varied and variable over time, even in a matter of few minutes, and contains elements which are not often found (e.g. tantalum) in particles of other origins. In this particular case, but the case is far from unique, the incinerator is located on a hill a few kilometres away from beaches which are very popular during the summer. Inevitably, the ash, light as it is, is carried by the wind and falls on the sand and into the sea.

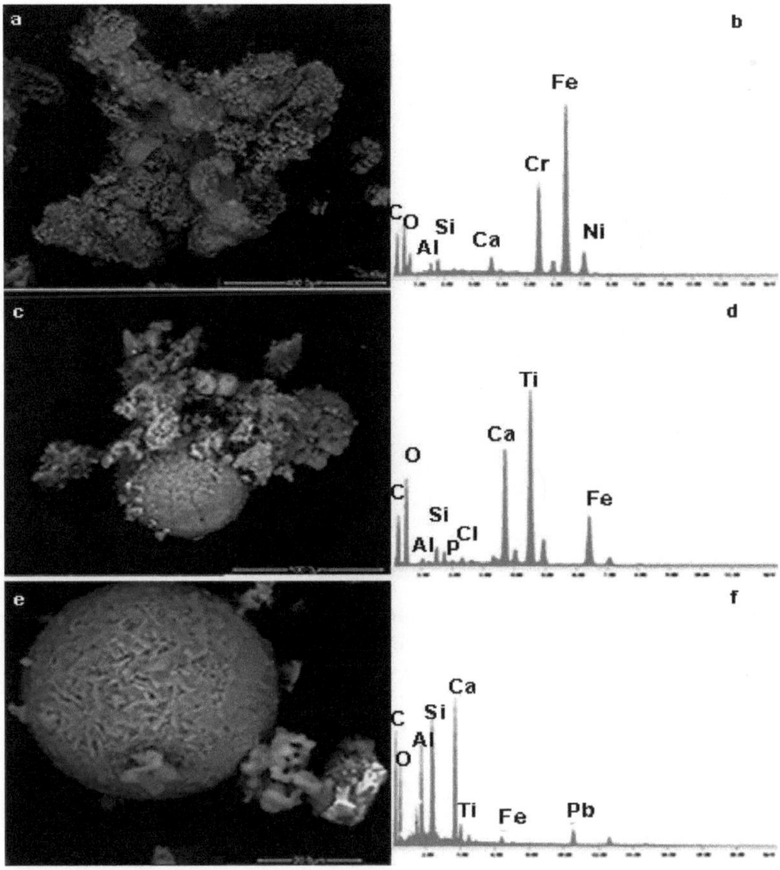

Figure 3.3 Ashes from an incinerator plant (Terni, Italy). The particles shown in the images belong to emissions from an incinerator plant located in a small Italian town and were collected in the air. The spherical shape with a surface made up of small juxtaposed crystals is typical of a high-temperature source. Very often other particles stick to larger ones when they are still hot and soft. Once cooled, the spherical particles, hollow inside, are very fragile and easily crumble, giving rise to particles which are obviously smaller and more numerous than the original ones. Steel, lead and titanium are the most common elements found in the environment.

The following images represent a selection of the dirtiness we inhale every day (Figs. 3.1–3.7).

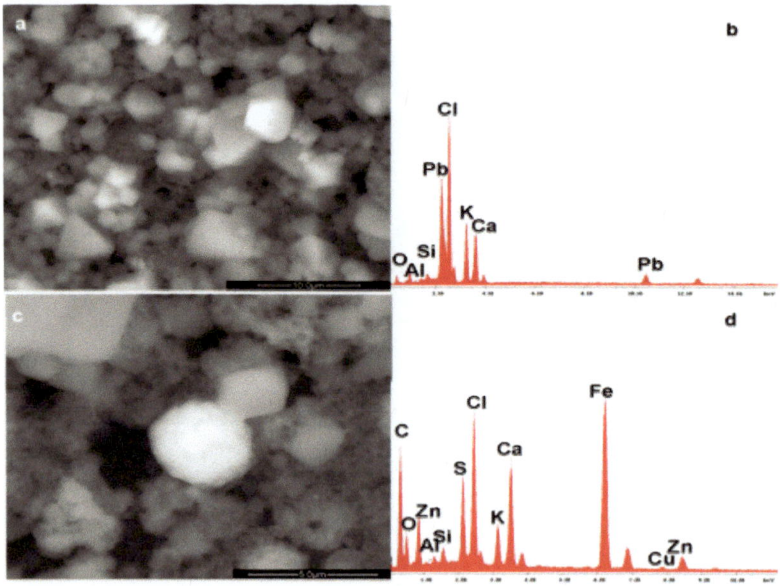

Figure 3.4 Dust from a waste incinerator plant. The particles shown in the images come from the storage placed below the combustion griddle of the municipal waste incinerator plant of a small town where two more waste incinerators are located. Similar particles are found everywhere in the area, on the ground, on any object or plant and suspended in the air.

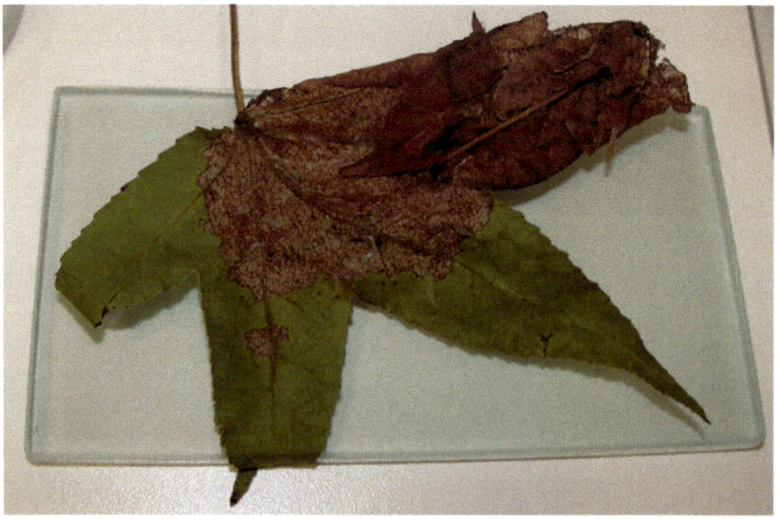

(a)

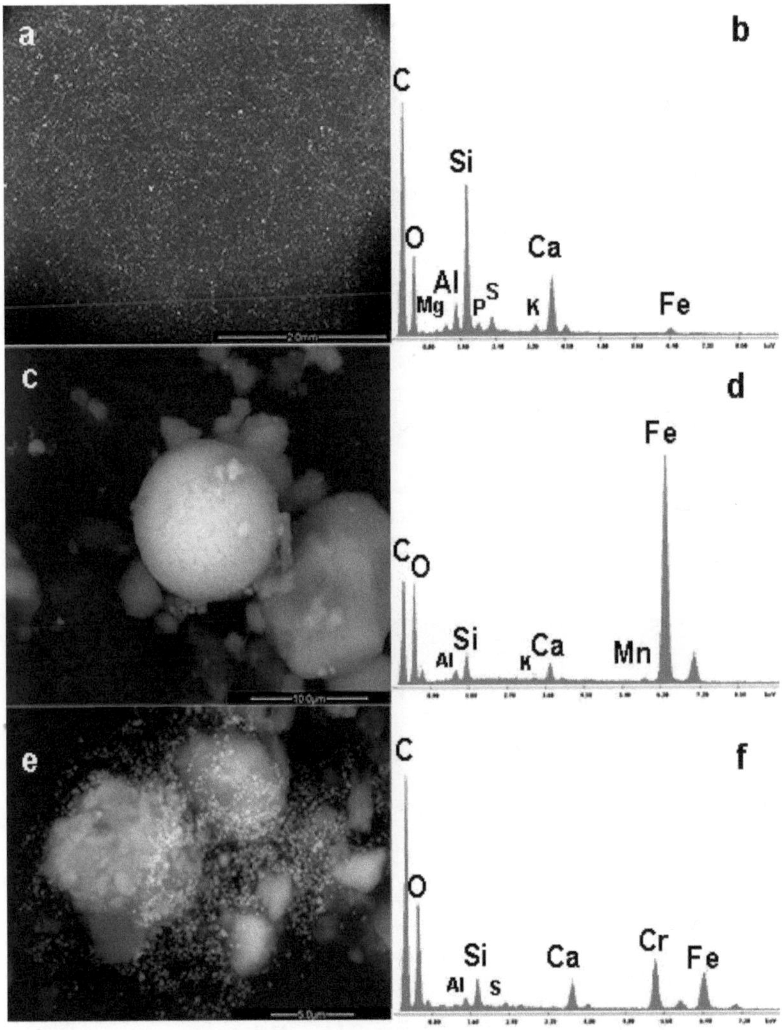

(b)

Figure 3.5 (a) A leaf damaged by waste incinerator emissions. Also the plants grown around incinerators are subjected to its pollution and can be severely damaged as this leaf demonstrates. The pollution identified on its surface is clearly related to the incinerator's emission. (b) The particles shown here were collected on leaves of plants grown in the outskirts of an industrial city, not far from a waste incinerator. The small particles are especially aggressive as they occlude the stomata of the leaves. The micro- and nanospherules are the result of high-temperature combustion. Elements like bismuth, iron and chromium were identified.

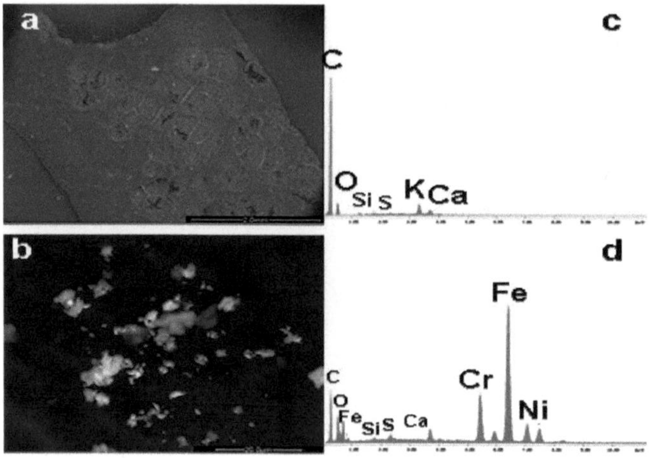

Figure 3.6 Leaf collected close to a waste incinerator plant. (a, b) The electron microscopy images refer to a leaf collected in the vicinity of a waste incinerator. (c) Elemental composition of the leaf. (d) Elemental composition (Fe-Cr-Ni, that is, steel) of some of the particles.

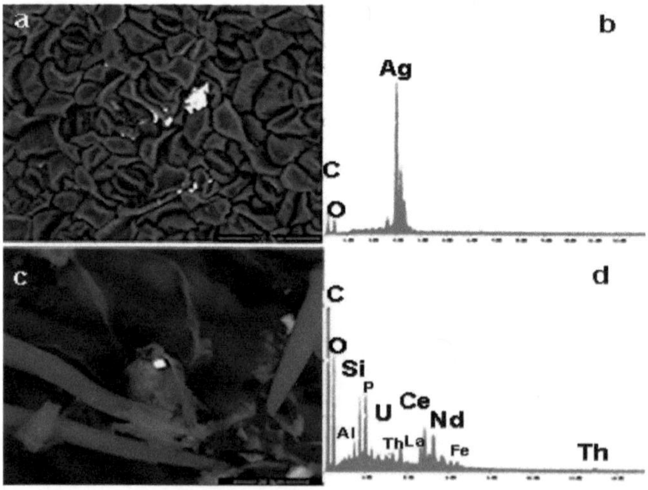

Figure 3.7 Leaf of a tree close to a ceramic factory. The particles shown were collected on leaves of plants grown in a glen at over 700 m altitude above sea level, far from inhabited centers. Wild vegetables grown in that place had fed for decades a person who then fell ill with peritoneal mesothelioma and eventually died of it. Note the composition of the particles containing thorium and uranium, two elements used as components of glazes by the small ceramic industries placed in a higher position, as the crow flies a couple of kilometres away from the glen, and with nothing standing in the way. We found also silver particles.

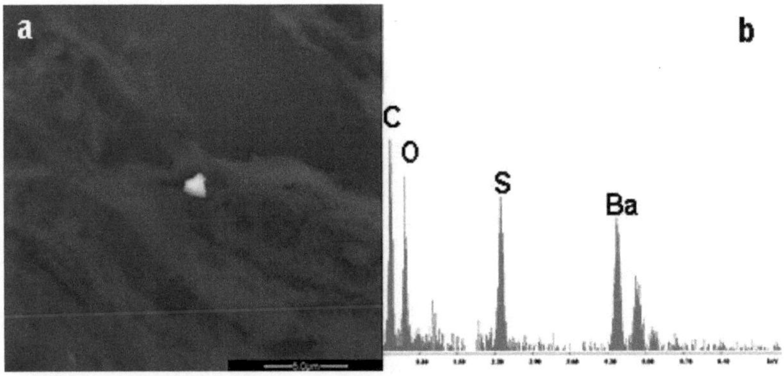

(a)

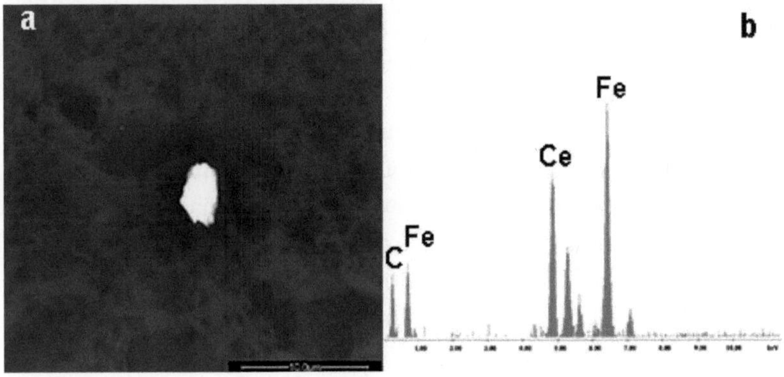

(b)

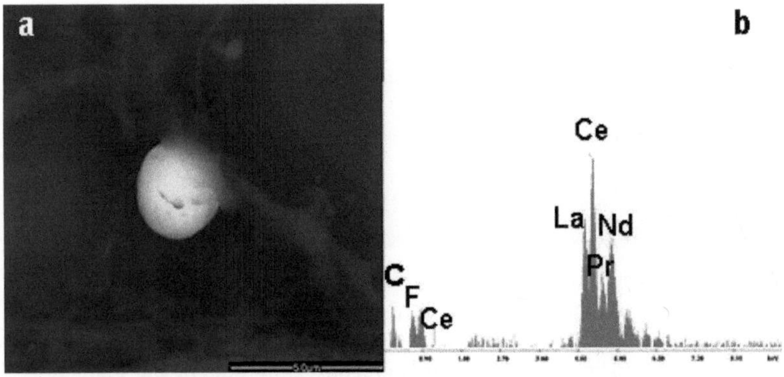

(c)

Figure 3.8 (a) Analysis of nose tissue affected by cancer in a patient living close to an incinerator plant. (b) Analysis of the nose cancer tissue. (c) Nose cancer. Basal cell carcinoma is the most common form of skin cancer. It is a papula or a slow-growing superficial nodule derived from some epidermal cells. They derive from keratinocytes close to the basal layer, which can be defined as basaloid keratinocytes. Metastases are not common, but untreated and let locally grow, they can destroy skin and bone. Barium-sulphur particles have been detected in this case. Barium sulphate is a very common salt used as a radiological contrast medium in the radiology of the digestive system. It can be used because it cannot be hydrolysed and, therefore, does not release barium ions, which are toxic. It is also often found in urban air pollution, resulting, among other origins, from the aging of buildings. Iron, cerium, lanthanum, neodymium and praseodymium are elements which can be very often found in smoking tobacco. Their particles are inhaled and breathed by smokers. In this case, it can be seen how, most likely, those particles crossed the alveolar barrier, were carried by the blood and ended up concentrating in the skin. One possible hypothesis is that the movement of the particles is an attempt by the organism to get rid of them without succeeding in going beyond the skin barrier.

If one considers them just from a chemical standpoint, nothing can be said about the biocompatibility of those pollutants, since they are substances which are not mentioned in specialised books and papers, and nobody tested their toxicity.

The following images (Fig. 3.8) show what was identified in the nose cancer of a person living in a house placed close to an urban waste incinerator plant.

The ash of the incinerators must be stored in landfills, but our politicians created laws in order to reuse them as fillers of cement or of asphalt.

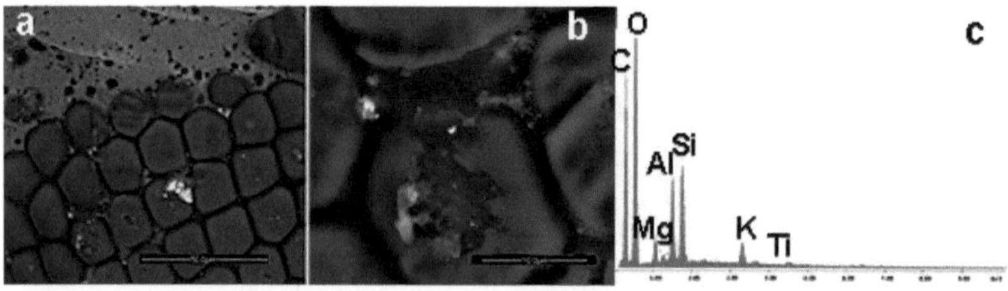

Figure 3.9 Insects, like all living things, are also attacked by particulate pollutants. The photographs show micro- and nanoparticles which have reached the eye of an ant. In this case, given the elemental chemical composition of the particles, it could be normal environmental dust generated by the soil.

Cement is not a material which is particularly capable of resisting time and bad weather. As for durability, its buildings can't be compared to those built centuries ago, which are still perfectly usable and accessible. Just as an example, there are still bridges and aqueducts built by the Romans about 20 centuries ago or more which are still used today. Consular roads such as, for example, the Via Emilia in Italy have not needed major maintenance for 2000 years. As a matter of fact, cement cannot last longer than a few decades. Yet, we keep using huge quantities of cement and we produce it in different varieties according to the particular intended use.

To make matters worse, now and for some time, most of the cements have been mixed with the ash left by the combustion of incinerators, thereby affecting their mechanical properties. This is undoubtedly one of the reasons why it is not unusual to see buildings and viaducts collapse in a time relatively close to their construction.

In addition, many cement plants operate as real waste incinerators and their mitigation systems concerning the dispersion of pollutants are much less effective than the already far-from-satisfactory ones used by waste incinerators.

We had a chance to carry out an investigation in a territory where grape-growing is the prevalent activity.

The analyses of the grape leaves (with which a famous sparkling wine is made) carried out in June showed the presence of copper sulphate currently used in agriculture and of calcium sulphate (cement) particles (Fig. 3.10).

3.3 Diesel Particulate Filter

As already reported, most solid, inorganic particulate matter produced by human activities is not degradable. The immediate consequence is that, as already mentioned, however little dust enters the environment, it will inevitably add to what is already present. In short, particles continue to accumulate.

Numerous sources of particulate matter are responsible for the situation, starting, as we already mentioned, from those of natural origin: volcanoes, rock and soil erosion, sand and forest fires, among others. On these causes it is actually impossible to intervene and take effective action. A different matter, however, is what regards the numerous anthropic sources: power plants operating with heavy oils and coal-fired biomass plants, domestic heating, waste incinerators, car traffic, etc. And car traffic is by far the easiest target.

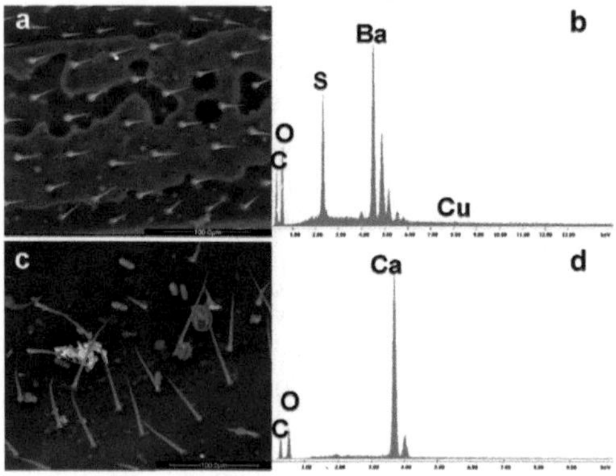
a
b
Ba
S
O
C
Cu
c
d
Ca
O
C

(a)

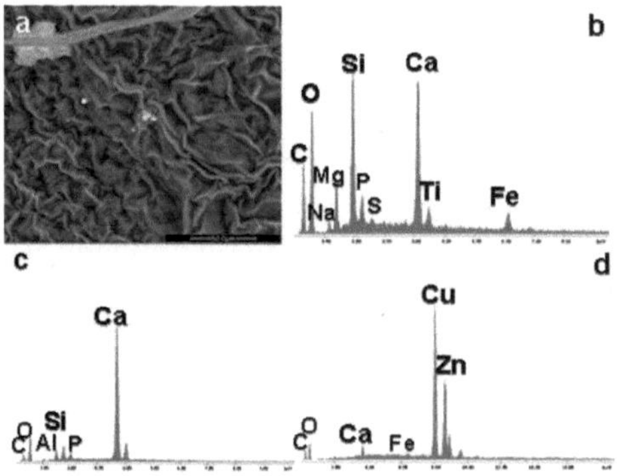
a
b
Si
Ca
O
C
Mg
P
Na
S
Ti
Fe
c
d
Ca
O
Si
C
Al
P
Cu
Zn
O
C
Ca
Fe

(b)

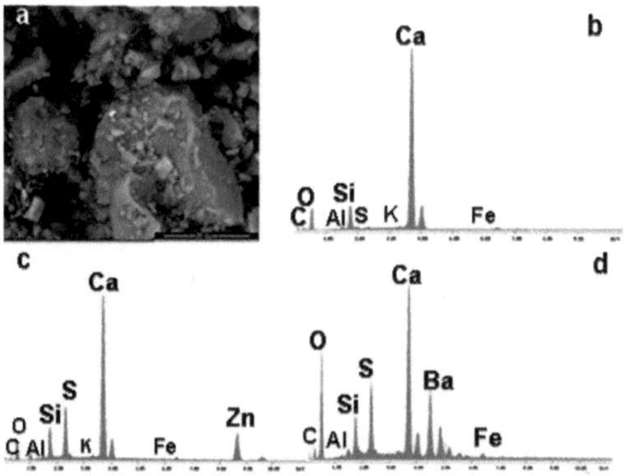
a
b
Ca
O
Si
C
Al
S
K
Fe
c
d
Ca
S
O
Si
C
Al
K
Fe
Zn
Ca
O
S
Ba
Si
C
Al
Fe

(c)

Figure 3.10 (a) Sample of a bee's body, contaminated. Particles expelled from the factory chimney were found on the whole body of the bees raised in the area surrounding the cement factory for a radius of a few kilometres. (b) Vine leaf contaminated. Particles fallen from the chimney of the cement factory containing those elements were found on the leaves of the vines and on the grapes collected within a radius of a few kilometres around the cement factory. (c) Cement. The images refer to a sample of Portland cement produced in an area where a type of grape is grown to produce a fine wine. Elements such as copper and zinc come from waste, which is treated at high temperature to be mixed with the finished product.

Diesel engines, in particular, produce considerable amounts of carbon particulate, and this is the cause of both strictly environmental and health problems.

In all advanced countries, there are maximum limits allowed for particle pollution (PM10 or PM2.5), and reaching and exceeding those limits is indicated by control units. What those control units do is weigh the amount of particles in relation to what is contained in a normal cubic metre (Nm^3) of air, that is, that volume of air measured under the standard conditions of 0°C and 1 atm of pressure. Diesel engines (but all internal combustion engines behave in the same way independently of the fuel) emit relatively coarse carbon particles, and once in the atmosphere, these are regularly weighed by the control units. So, to not incur penalties, it is expedient to make sure that the control units detect a weight which is as small as possible.

The simplest way to do this is to burn the carbonaceous particles so as to transform them into gases which, obviously, preserve the mass but which, on earth, do not have a weight, that is, a value detectable by a scale. In this way the control units, in fact scales, will not detect anything.

This is what a diesel particulate filter (DPF) does, burning the particles captured inside a device located along the exhaust pipe downstream of the engine (Fig. 3.11).

Leaving aside the obvious conservation of mass, that is, something which does not depend on human will, the major problem is that of the content of the captured particles. They are made of carbonaceous material, but each of them contains smaller particles of metallic nature derived from the friction of the mechanical parts (piston and cylinder) and from the additives which are components of fuels and lubricants. Those metal particles cannot be burned, are emitted into the atmosphere and are preserved as such wherever they end up. Being contained in the coarse carbon-based particle, they are obviously smaller and more numerous than their original containers and, therefore, they are more aggressive towards health than are the untreated emissions.

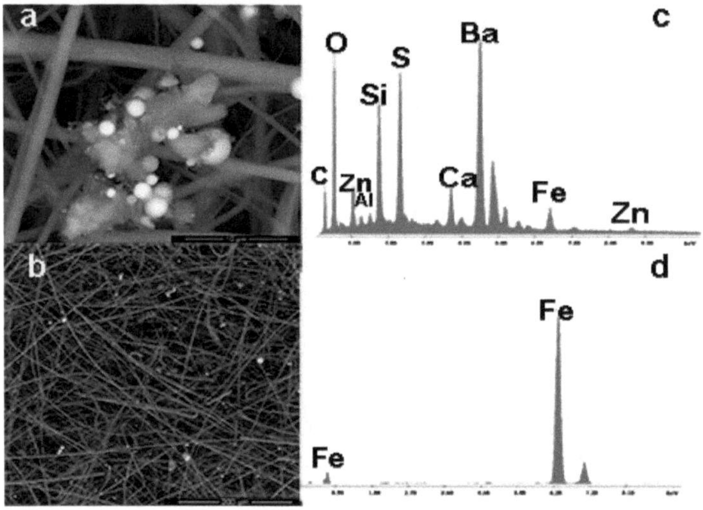

Figure 3.11 DPF. The filaments seen in the electron microscopy images are those of the filter on which the exhaust gases of an automobile equipped with a DPF were collected for our analysis. The numerous particles captured by our filter would not have been freed from their carbon matrix into the environment if the anti-particulate device had not burned it, turning it into carbon oxides. As often mentioned, the spherical shape is characteristic of high-temperature formation. In the image at higher magnification it can be seen how part of the carbonaceous matrix (grey and formless around the particles) remains unburned.

In the book *Nanopathology: The Health Impact of Nanoparticles* (Pan Stanford Publishing 2008, now Jenny Stanford Publishing, page 212), we showed that the filters we checked emitted in the environment cerium dioxide used in the system and nanoparticles of platinum present as a catalytic converter. It should be added that while some DPFs use cerium dioxide to trigger the combustion of carbon particles at a relatively low temperature, others use ferrocene, an organo-metallic compound consisting of two cyclopentadienyl rings linked on opposite sides of a central iron atom, which cannot fail to enter the atmosphere – two substances whose toxicity has never been thoroughly studied and which would certainly not have been released into the atmosphere without the use of those systems. In conclusion, the DPF system is presented as a technical means to avoid pollution so much that it has become mandatory in diesel vehicles but which, in fact, like it or not, is a producer of aggressive particles.

3.4 War and Terrorism

There can be no doubt: war is made to kill or, in any case, to cause damage to the enemy. It is not always certain, however, that those damages, so desired and achieved by expenditure of energy and money as they are, are made only to those against whom a war is being fought.

When, centuries ago, the armies began to use explosives, the inevitable side effect was that of generating clouds of dust, and dust is never beneficial, no matter by which side it is produced.

Over time, as happens with industrial technologies, also in warfare combustion, temperatures keep growing higher and higher, and as we already know, the higher they are, the finer the dust generated is, with all its consequences on the environment and on people's health.

Modern wars pollute the environment like never before with wars of the past, and many examples could be made.

It is normal for civilian settlements to be destroyed and at least partially reduced to dust, but strategic objectives are the favourite targets, many of which are polluting establishments as such. Bombs against strategic targets such as weapons factories, chemical factories or power plants lead to a very particular increase of the pollution of the area, pollution which, generally, is not monitored if not, and certainly not always, at the end of the war, but which continues to exist often for a long time when peace has been restored and which, because of the mobility of pollutants, can also involve neighbouring countries which had not been part in the conflict.

In 1999, the Pancevo (Serbia) refinery was bombed for three consecutive days. Aside from the civilians who died immediately, the tanks of unrefined oil went to fire and produced a tall column of toxic fumes. As the cloud carried by the wind was heading towards the US base, the American planes took off and scattered silver iodide particles to cause rain according to a well-known technique. The rain, rich in silver iodide particles mixed with the soot produced by the combustion of the oil, a soot containing bromide-chlorine-lead particles, contaminated the pastures and the river Danube, which flows into the Black Sea.

The extent of such damage is very difficult to assess, but to be sure, as often happens in similar cases, there is not even the will to do it.

Figure 3.12 shows an example of a post-mortem finding of nanoparticles (10 nm) dispersed in the lymph nodes of an inhabitant of Pancevo who died of lymphoma in the university hospital of Sarajevo. The soot of the combustion of the unrefined oil was detected in his corpse.

It must be remembered that in the course of the fighting involving Kuwait and Iraq, several oil wells were set on fire, becoming for a time enormous sources of pollution with all the consequences of the case.

And other pollution, albeit of lesser proportions and with consequences almost only to the detriment of the soldiers closely involved, was due to the destruction of weapons captured by the enemy, making them explode.

It is not at all surprising that after the end of the conflicts, cancer pathologies began to appear with a particularly high frequency with civilians, while the first victims were the soldiers. The longer-term consequences, however, are borne by the inhabitants of the areas involved, where pollution is inevitably destined to remain for a time which is hard to predict but, in any case, will be very long and will also affect generations to come. It is a fact that the observatory founded in Sarajevo after the end of the Balkan War continues today to record an increase in cancer cases which would have been unexpected if the conflict had not existed. As is obvious, cancer and other pathologies related to war pollution do not spare those who have fled the conflict zones, and therefore, one can die of war even far in space and time from it.

Of the pathologies linked to the wars fought in the Persian Gulf and in the Balkans, there is no exhaustive news, because not a little has been kept hidden and continues to be so. For example, little or nothing is known about what happened to many soldiers of the NATO forces.

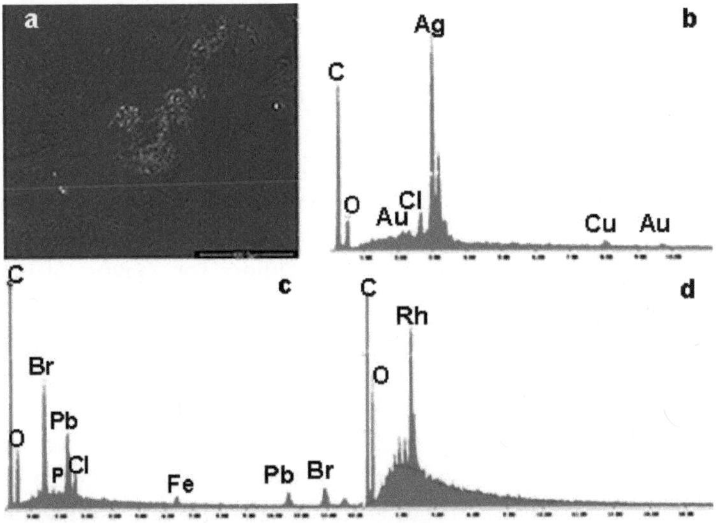

Figure 3.12 War lymphoma case from Pancevo. Lymphoma is a form of cancer we have come across most often by analysing pathological findings of both soldiers and non-military subjects active in the territories where a war was being fought or had been fought in the past and of inhabitants of those areas. In war environments, the concentration of particles can be very high, and it happens that large quantities of dust enter the body quickly and repeatedly. Macrophages intervene massively before the particles are enveloped by granulation tissue and move them to the lymph nodes where, being non-biodegradable and impossible to eliminate, they remain and give rise to cancer of the lymphatic system. Typically, cancer needs a long-enough time to manifest itself, and therefore, many cases have become evident after the war had ended for years. The fact must also be considered that the non-degradability of the particles and, therefore, their remaining unchanged in the environment extend their pathogenicity for a long time. The elemental analysis highlights the complex composition of the particles of war origin, a composition which is not found in 'normal' urban pollution and which is due to high-temperature explosions involving the most disparate materials.

Apparently, the Gulf Wars have affected American and British soldiers the most, while those of the Balkans seem to have affected Italians more, although there are certainly cases of other nationalities.

The pathologies look quite similar, although it seems that the American soldiers have suffered from neurological problems with psychiatric implications much more than has happened to the Italian soldiers with whom we have dealt most.

Some explanations for these differences could be sought in the fact that in the wars fought in the Persian Gulf numerous oil wells were set on fire and a large amount of armaments, perhaps even chemical in nature, were destroyed by making them explode so as not to have to bring them to the United States.

It is also necessary to take into account the medicaments, some of which lacking adequate testing and, in any case, without any authorisation to trade, taken by US soldiers (or, maybe, of other nationalities?) to prevent possible attacks by chemical weapons carried out by the enemy army. Of those drugs, their side effects and their mutual interactions, there is not enough information to express any judgment. Often there is no information at all.

Terrorism, particularly modern one, is much subtler than traditional war and, in a way, is harder to understand and to face, as it follows a logic which is at least partially different from what is 'reasonable' and definitely unusual. But, regardless of considerations which can't be part of this discussion, there are instances, as was the case of the attack on the Twin Towers in New York, where the medium- and long-term consequences from the health point of view are absolutely similar.

3.4.1 Depleted-Uranium Weapons

In the 1970s depleted uranium (DU) started being secretly experimented in weapons, and some years later it was actively used.

Uranium is a metal belonging to the actinide series of the periodic table with 92 protons and as many electrons, of which 6 are valence electrons. All its isotopes are unstable, and for that reason, uranium is weakly radioactive.

Isotope U238 with its 146 neutrons is by far the most common in nature, accounting for about 99.3% of the whole quantity. Isotope U235 (143 neutrons) accounts for almost all the rest, since the other isotopes (only U234 among them is natural, while the others, 232, 233 and 236, are produced artificially in breeder reactors from U235 and thorium) are extremely rare.

Both industry (nuclear plants) and war (nuclear bombs) exploit the unique properties of U235, it being the only fissile isotope of a natural element, that is, capable of sustaining a nuclear chain reaction with neutrons at any energy. For that reason, U235 is extracted from the whole mass of natural uranium, which, because of that, at the end of the process is 'depleted', while the uranium meant to be used for industrial or military applications to which U235 is added is 'enriched' in its isotope. It should be specified that the civil use of uranium requires a much lower enrichment than that required for the manufacture of nuclear weapons.

What is left from the process of depletion and the comparatively very small amount of DU produced by recycling nuclear fuel has a much lower value and is used, also combined with titanium, sandwiched between two sheets of steel in tank amour plates, to make shielding of industrial radiography cameras, as counterbalance weights in aircraft wings, as ballast in boats, as a counterweight in elevators, as a chemical catalyst, to colour glass, to make ceramic glaze and, until not a very long time ago, even in dentistry to give false teeth a more 'natural' look [1, 2].

But uranium – in this case, technically speaking, depleted or whole makes no difference – has some characteristics which make it fit to be used in projectiles. First of all, being a waste, it is relatively inexpensive, then it is heavy (its density is about 19.1 g/cm^3), non-brittle (unlike, for example, tungsten, another metal used in armaments) and an excellent penetrator because at the condition of impact with the target it is 'self-sharpening' (adiabatic shear). The most relevant feature as to pollution, though, is its being pyrophoric, that is, liable to ignite spontaneously on exposure to air, when thinly sliced or reduced to powder. A relatively small volume of uranium inserted in a shell can produce a temperature exceeding 3000°C at the target hit, a temperature and an amount of heat high enough to have much of what has been struck evaporate. As happens in waste incinerators, and a fortiori because of the more extreme conditions, much of the matter is reduced to small molecules or, much more often, to atoms which are thrown away from the impact spot and, reaching quickly a colder environment, recombine into solid particles whose composition is totally random.

The presence of uranium – though, of course, present in the phenomenon – is extremely rare in the particles generated or, in fact, is absent at all because of its very small amount as compared with the rest of the materials and because of its heavy weight, a feature which makes it fall quickly and after a comparatively short trip and stay in the air. As a matter of fact, uranium particles can be found only in the immediate surroundings of the explosion, as can be seen from the US document 'Air Force Exploratory Development Project 06CD0101' about experiments with DU projectiles which were carried out between October 1977 and October 1978 at the military base of Eglin (Florida). That document is particularly interesting because it makes clear that the military scientists who worked on the project, though lacking direct experience on humans, had already understood what the danger is with regards to health when such an armament is used.

Like any micro- and, especially, nanoparticles, those produced by DU explosions stay for some time suspended in the air, fall to the ground, are often lifted again by the wind and move in the atmosphere also along considerable distances while their concentration obviously decreases. But concentration close to the impact spot, also because of the occasional frequency of the explosion in a relatively small territory, is often particularly high, and soldiers, Red Cross and humanitarian workers and, in general, people present there inhale great quantities of those pollutants besides ingesting them with food.

Conditions, particularly due to the small size of the particles, are such that the typical pathological situations induced by fine and ultrafine particles are established quickly. In fact, a particularly high number of soldiers deployed in territories where war was being, or had been, waged are repatriated ill or become ill soon after. Local people, who are supposed to be at least as ill as soldiers, are very hard to control because of the unfavourable conditions they live in, and most of the information which leaks comes from journalists or personnel of non-governmental organisations (NGOs) active in those areas. Nothing properly collected and sorted, and in particular, nothing reliable comes from official data.

In our laboratory we had a chance to analyse the biopsic and post-mortem pathological samples of about 330 soldiers, and only in one of them could we find trace of uranium in particulate form: a rarity which was expected for the reasons just explained. What we generally see are great quantities of particles, in many cases agglomerated nanoparticles whose composition is varied and whose shape is either spherical, as is typical of high-temperature generation or, particularly in the larger findings, geometrically irregular as is the case with shards of big spherical particles or particles generated at the margin of the phenomenon, which is, in areas where temperature is colder.

What happens with DU can happen with any other armament sharing similar features. Tungsten, for example, is a pyrophoric element also used in weapons with the 'advantage' of reaching a temperature around 5000°C, though it is much less popular than uranium because of both technical and economical drawbacks.

Years ago, the problem with soldiers being repatriated ill from war theaters with then unknown sets of symptoms came almost immediately to the fore, and several alleged perpetrators was indicated by various sources.

As mentioned, cocktails of drugs were usually administered to soldiers, in particular before starting to serve in the assigned territory, but each country had its own recipes, recipes which were not even the same within the same national army, and it is not sure that all soldiers had been subjected to treatment. Vaccines (of which little is known) had been blamed, a thesis which has certainly some reasons to exist, given the number and variety of vaccinations out of any control soldiers underwent in very short periods of time. Then as now, their bodies were not allowed the necessary time to recover from the collection of stimuli received. Then as now, no attention was given to the possible presence of allergy against drug components. Then as now, nobody even bothered to establish whether the subject was naturally immune against one or more diseases against which he was vaccinated, a precaution which Napoleonic doctors applied in 1805 when they introduced the smallpox vaccination in the army, but which seems to be unknown today. But also journalist, NGO staff and local people manifested the same symptoms without having been vaccinated or having taken particular medications. So, vaccines and drugs could be accepted, at most, as contributory causes facilitating the triggering of pathologies. For a short time, also chemicals sprayed on some of the tents groups of soldiers slept in were brought up, but the vast majority of sufferers had never spent a moment in those tents. Not to say of the ill civilians. When the use of DU armament was admitted after having been denied for years, uranium was also blamed as a toxic and radioactive element. Some traces were actually found in the urine of soldiers, but no radioactivity was detected in their pathological tissues. As a matter of fact, uranium is by no means a rare element, being more abundant than iodine, selenium, cadmium, silver, etc. It is roughly as common as tin and zinc, and some can be found in drinking water and in vegetables, particularly in their roots, grown in soil where it is contained (e.g. granite weathering soils) or where some polluted mineral phosphorous fertilisers are used. According to Anke et al. [3], 'The uranium content of 116 foodstuffs and beverages varies extremely. Vegetable foods accumulate between 0.8 μg U/kg dry matter (DM) in margarine, bee honey and pearl barley, 50 μg U/kg DM in asparagus, and >100 μg U/kg DM in mixed mushrooms. As a rule, sugar-, starch- and fat-rich foodstuffs proved to be uranium-poor (fruits, seeds, flour), whereas leafy vegetables, tea and herbs can be uranium-rich. Animal foodstuffs accumulate lower uranium contents, with 0.7 μg U/kg DM in butter and 1.1–1.9 μg U/kg DM in condensed and normal cow's milk, 1.5–3.1 μg U/kg DM in pork, beef, chicken and mutton, 3–10 μg U/kg DM in fish, and 16 μg U/kg DM in hen's eggs.' So, finding traces of uranium in the urine is by no means surprising and is also proof that the organism, unlike what happens with particles, can eliminate it. As to radioactivity and its effects, it must be noted that the technical staff working in the preparation of uranium weapons, and therefore in constant contact with that metal, never showed any signs of disease.

Particles are the only pathogen shared equally by all people who spent or spend their time in war theaters and are the only pathogen which can be found in all patients. So, all other harmful agents more or less frequently present in the territories or in the situations involving those pathologies can be regarded, at most, as contributory causes.

In conclusion, if a sort of court ruling should be issued, finding no trace of uranium but the clear traces of its activity, uranium would be, all considered, not the actual killer but the 'guy behind'.

It may be interesting to observe that probably the most common symptom shared by all sick soldiers is chronic fatigue, a condition we find almost invariably in all patients affected by nanopathologies. Sometimes, the symptom is treated with cortisone drugs which have an effect which is that of doping in sports. Ultimately, not a cure but a palliative not to see the symptom. Other common symptoms are irritability, insomnia and the loss of primary (or short-term) memory, that is, the capacity of holding information in mind for a short period of time (e.g. to remember a telephone number which has been just communicated.) In most cases, those symptoms are attributed to post-traumatic stress, something the Mayo Clinic defines as 'a mental health condition that's triggered by a terrifying event – either experiencing it or witnessing it. Symptoms may include flashbacks, nightmares and severe anxiety, as well as uncontrollable thoughts about the event.'

In almost all cases, the disorder is dealt with several, often combined, types of psychotherapy, but particularly with soldiers, the treatment is usually made through anti-depressant and anti-anxiety medications. Far from us the intention to criticise the usefulness of these therapies aimed at treating the shocking effects of war experience, but, though having assets of only few hundreds of cases analysed, we have had patients suffering from those symptoms which were nothing else but the result of particles later found in the brain after having triggered a cancer. It is possible that a more complete diagnosis would have allowed to implement a more appropriate and timely treatment than psychoactive drugs alone.

It is only natural that the behaviour of the micro- and nanoparticles we deal with is the same in soldiers as in any individual. So, the nanopathologies are basically the same. The main difference lies in the speed with which these become clinically evident in soldiers, and this because of the large quantities of dust, composed especially of ultrafine particles, to which they are exposed together with very complex combinations of other toxic substances.

It can be interesting to point out that, as a rule, the soldiers sent to war zones are young and leave in health conditions comparable to those of an athlete.

Our case history of war-related illnesses counts about 330 cases divided into cases of Hodgkin's and non-Hodgkin's lymphoma, leukaemia and cancer of different parts of the body (the lung, the liver, the kidneys, the brain, the thyroid, the colon, the stomach and cases of blood disorders). As already reported, we did not find uranium in the samples analysed (except in one case, and we have no evidence that uranium came from a bomb) but found evident traces of the war-field pollution generated by high-technology weapons against specific targets (tanks, metallurgical and chemist factories, etc.) (Fig. 3.13).

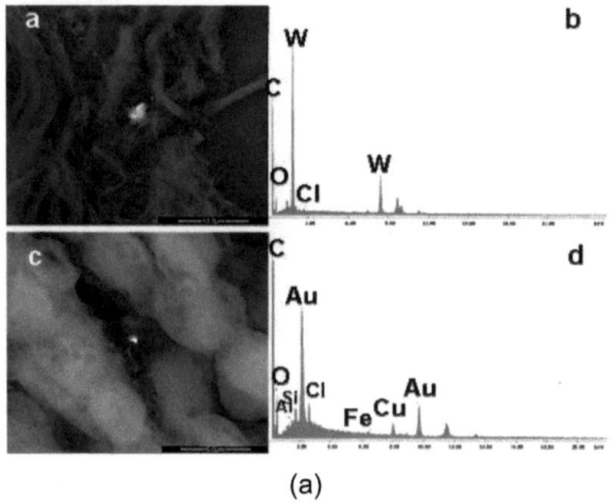

Figure 3.13 (a and b) Images of two cases of soldiers affected by lymphoma. (b) Lymphoma of a soldier.

In about 330 cases of soldiers with cancer whose biopsy or autopsy findings we have analysed, lymphoma is by far the most frequent variety. In all cases, solid, inorganic and non-biodegradable micro- and nanoparticles were present in the analysed tissues as is the case here shown by electron microscopy photographs and energy-dispersive X-ray spectroscopy (EDS) graphs. Stainless steel (iron-chromium-nickel), titanium and tungsten are elements which are commonly found in this type of finding. It is not uncommon to find gold, an element used for war purposes, as a component.

One of the authors of this book, Dr. Gatti, had the opportunity as a member of the Italian Governmental Commissions (2004–12) on 'Depleted Uranium and Related Diseases' and as a member of the scientific committee on the 'Prevention and Control of the Illnesses of the Soldiers' (CPCM) to investigate also in an international firing range and on the people living around the military area. She had the chance to analyse the bones of a shepherd who died of leukaemia whose body was exhumed after 10 years from death (Fig. 3.14).

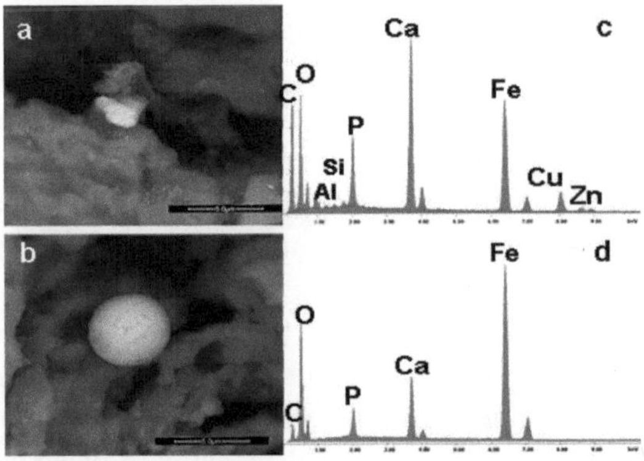

Figure 3.14 Bone marrow analyses of an exhumed body affected by leukaemia. The particles shown in the electron microscopy images were found in the bone marrow remains of a corpse exhumed several years after burial. The corpse is that of a young shepherd who died of leukaemia who lived in the territory of a large military shooting range where explosive weapons are tested. As we have seen in quite a few other cases, not only soldiers but also civilians living in the area affected by pollution are ill with war-related nanopathologies. Unlike other pollutants, especially if of organic origin, which can be transformed over time after inhumation until they disappear completely, non-biodegradable, solid, inorganic particles are preserved indefinitely, and their detection can be used as a marker of a pollution condition. Calcium and phosphorus are components of the bone tissue, while elements like iron, copper and zinc are due to pollution. The spherical particle was obviously generated at high temperature.

3.5 The Case of the World Trade Center

On 18 September 2001, a week after the attacks to the Twin Towers and the Pentagon, Christie Whitman, administrator of the US Environmental Protection Agency (EPA) announced that air and drinking water had been monitored both in New York and in

Washington and they were 'safe', adding, 'We are very encouraged that the results from our monitoring of air quality and drinking water conditions in both New York and near the Pentagon show that the public in these areas is not being exposed to excessive levels of asbestos or other harmful substances.' The document continues describing briefly how the monitoring had been carried out and what clean-up measures had been adopted [4, 5].

Almost a couple of decades later, the extent of the disaster is not yet clear, but it involves in a chronic way the heath of many hundreds of thousands of people who inhaled and ingested the fine and ultrafine dust created by the collapse the two aircraft aerosolised and the very high temperature of the phenomenon. In early 2020, at the time of writing these pages, three more firefighters, who began to get sick after six months of working at Ground Zero, died of the cancer they had started to develop after their exposure to the dust.

Among the enormous variety of materials contained in the two aircraft and in the two buildings there were huge quantities of asbestos, and those mineral nanofibres were transformed by the heat into something even smaller and, therefore, more penetrating. Generally, mesothelioma, the typical asbestos-induced cancer, takes a long time, often decades, to become clinically visible. Yet, some people who were involved in the disaster have already died of it.

Unfortunately, but, from a certain point of view, understandably, a lot of people flocked to the disaster site immediately after its occurrence: firefighters, the police and health rescuers, trying to do something to rescue non-existing survivors. But there were also journalists, photographers, medical staff and common people curious to see what had happened. Many, in particular firefighters and the police, returned for months to Ground Zero. All of them, regardless of their job and the reason why they were there, submitted themselves to a huge risk. But that dust spread over a very large area, and even those who had not approached the scene of the disaster but, however, lived in the New York area were inevitably affected [5].

So, 9/11, whoever those responsible were, was the first terrorist attack on a massive scale and was much more successful in terms of damage inflicted than the perpetrators themselves had expected.

We had the possibility to analyse the dust deposited on the work uniform of a firefighter, a dusty object taken from a shop which was located inside the Twin Towers and the sweat of some firefighters who underwent a special treatment of decontamination one year after their contamination.

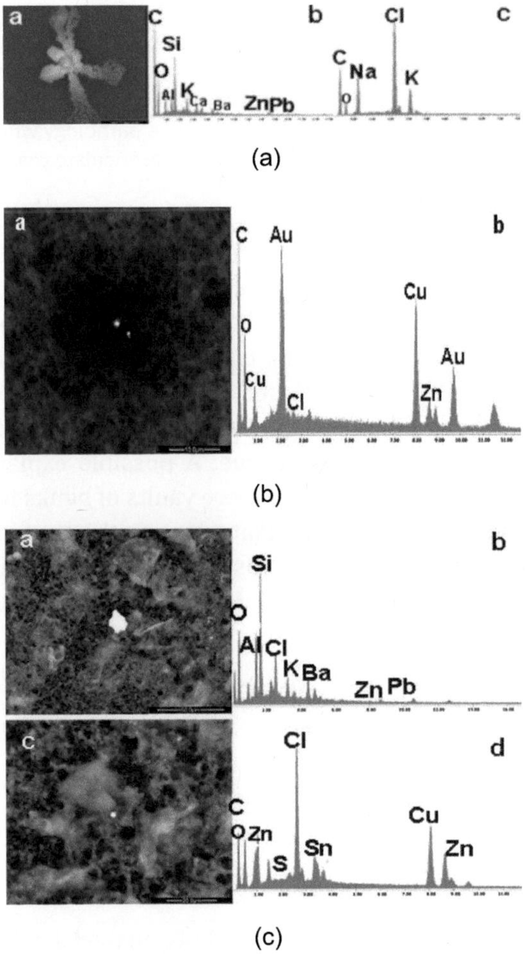

Figure 3.15 (a) Firefighter's sweat. (b) Firefighter's sweat contamination. The electron microscopy photographs (a and b) show some particles detected in the sweat, dark in colour, of firefighters who worked immediately after the collapse of the Twin Towers in New York in what is now called Ground Zero. The sweat collection was carried out four years after the exposure of the subjects and still contained evident traces of the dust which could have been breathed and swallowed and that the organism, it is not known how effectively, was expelling through the sweat. The detected particles are similar to those found on objects and clothing which were hit by the dust caused by the collapse. It is not possible

(*Continued*)

to determine, however, whether the particles found in the analyses shown in the images actually date back to what entered the body of the firefighters while they were working in 2011 or if, instead, they are particles still present in New York which entered the body later, in a moment temporally close to that of the production of sweat. The composition of those particles is extremely varied and complex, and this is due to the complexity of the structure and content of the collapsed buildings and the two aircraft which were reduced to dust of all sizes. (c) Sweat of a female patient suffering from a pathology which was never clearly diagnosed but who was contaminated by particulate matter contained particles as well.

The sweat contained some particles whose chemical composition could be related to the dust originated by the event. In our already quoted book *Nanopathology* (page 255), there are some examples of particulate matter identified. The composition is unusual and does not correspond to any known material: for example, particles of gold alloyed with zinc and tin were identified in the sweat, and they were also incorporated in the fatty tissue. A possible explanation was that inside the Twin Towers there were vaults of banks hosting gold bars which were melted by the heat, along with other metals, thus forming odd particulate which was immediately dispersed in the environment (Fig. 3.15).

3.6 Engineered Nanoparticles and Nanotechnologies

Unlike the great majority of particles, only some of them, but increasingly, are expressly manufactured in specialised laboratories.

Their synthesis can take place in two different ways, called top-down and bottom-up.

Top-down synthesis starts from bulk material whose size is progressively reduced by attrition or milling. In the bottom-up approach, the particles are made by self-assembly as happens, for instance, with chemical synthesis [6].

Actually, particles are not only an undesirable side effect: when they are designed and manufactured in a targeted manner by a specialised laboratory, they are something of whose extraordinary properties, unexpected until a few decades ago, interesting technical and financial advantage can be taken. In fact, the investments in this field are huge and on the increase.

Nanoparticles have unique physical and chemical properties which, in many respects, are very different from those of the same compositions in the bulk. At the nanoscale, materials behave very differently compared to the same materials at larger scales and it is not easy to predict with sufficient accuracy those properties when applied to a single particle. Colour may change (in function of their size), and so electrical conductance, wettability and many other properties. As a matter of fact, the chemical processes taking place on the surfaces of nanoparticles are very complicated and, for the time being, remain largely unknown. Only with direct experience can reliable information be obtained. Which, moreover, is valid for all science proper.

All that has been briefly explained so far must be considered when it comes to evaluating the action of nanoparticles within biological tissues. Too little is known about this, and often even the little which is known is overlooked.

The phenomena making nanoparticles different from the bulk version of the same material are mainly based on 'quantum effects' and the high ratio between surface and volume. Nanoscale materials have a much larger surface area than an equal mass of larger-scale material, and as surface area per mass of a material grows larger, a greater amount of it can come into contact with the surrounding matter, that way increasing reactivity. Most biological processes occur at the nanoscale, and their observation gives scientists and technologists models and templates to imagine and construct new processes which find application in medicine, imaging, computing, printing, chemistry (chemical catalysis in particular or, to be more accurate, the supply of energy necessary to have a certain reaction occur, which is not catalysis proper), synthesis of new materials and many other applications in what is called nanotechnology.

It is necessary to know that all laboratory processes related to the production of nanoparticles are potentially risky for operators. In fact, they can come into continuous contact with the particles, and therefore, it is advisable to work in suitable environmental conditions, including positive pressure.

A practical problem which is not always easy to solve when working with nanoparticles is their strong tendency to attract each other.

The mutual attraction can determine two different situations: one called clustering, in which the particles joined together can be separated through an ultrasound treatment, and the other called aggregation, where the situation is irreversible and it is no longer possible to return to the starting point, that is, of single particles.

So, engineered nanoparticles are very hard to handle, and among other technical problems, this makes it difficult to carry out biological experiments, particularly in vivo ones, as the investigators think they are administering nanoparticles to their subject (generally cells or an animal), while what they actually deal with are much larger entities, and those larger entities produce results which cannot be those of nanoparticles, the volume of which differs by several orders of magnitude. Therefore, it can happen that some results reported in the literature as due to nanoparticles are actually those of microparticles.

A further problem is the ease with which different metal nanoparticles tend to ignite when handled at room temperature and in a normal air atmosphere due to their high surface-to-volume ratio and, as a consequence, their great energy.

Engineered particles are at the base of nanotechnologies, that is, one of the biggest financial investments in the history of economy. If it is true that particles give very advantageous properties to the products, it is equally true that, as is almost normally the case in industry, the entire life cycle of the object which is being designed or actually manufactured is too rarely taken into due consideration. In this case, the first safety problem to be addressed is that relating to production conditions, and then comes the contact of the product with the user. But the main problem is how to dispose of the product once, whatever the reason, it is no longer needed. Although not always, in most cases, the particles used are almost indestructible, and in one way or another, they will end up in the environment, where they will accumulate with those already present.

Nowadays they are used to make new products now commercially available, like clothes, paints, computer and telephone parts, pesticides, deodorants, drugs, etc., growing more and more popular. Nevertheless, it should be clarified that to date, the quantity of the engineered nanoparticles present on earth is far smaller than that of the particles of natural origin and those of unintentional anthropic origin. Still, they are growing contributors to pollution.

3.7 How Particles Behave in the Environment

It is a matter of fact that once particles come out of their origin, for example, the chimney stack of an incinerator, as already mentioned, they travel and reach distances which can be enormous. As an already mentioned example, the grains of sand in the Sahara Desert, far coarser than the particles we deal with, reach the eastern shores of the United States, where we found them. It is equally clear that the smaller the particle volume, the greater the distance it reaches. It is also this aspect which the various diffusion models should take into particular account. Therefore, if the fallout map must be reliable, in addition to considering many other aspects, including those related to weather events, it is essential to know the composition of the particles with respect to their mass.

Another important aspect of the characteristic behaviour of the particles once they have fallen to the ground is the fact of penetrating, especially dragged by the rain, into the aquifers, polluting them. But they also change the composition of the soil, for example, because of what is released as a result of corrosion. This changes the habitat of the microflora and the microfauna with consequences which are often hard to predict. A notable phenomenon is their possible interference with the root system of plants (Fig. 3.16).

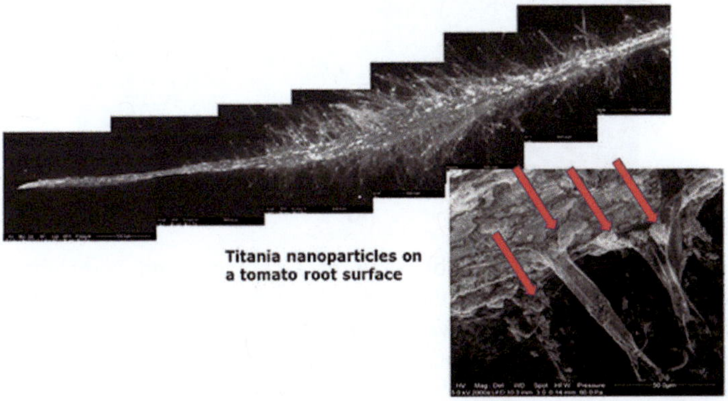

Figure 3.16 Tomato roots with nanoparticles. Scanning electron microscopy image of a root of a tomato plant immersed in a solution of water with 500 mg/l of nanoparticles of TiO_2 (INESE–IIT-Project 2009–2013). The arrows indicate a cluster of nanoparticles of TiO_2 which occlude the pores of the roots, hindering the adsorption of nutrients.

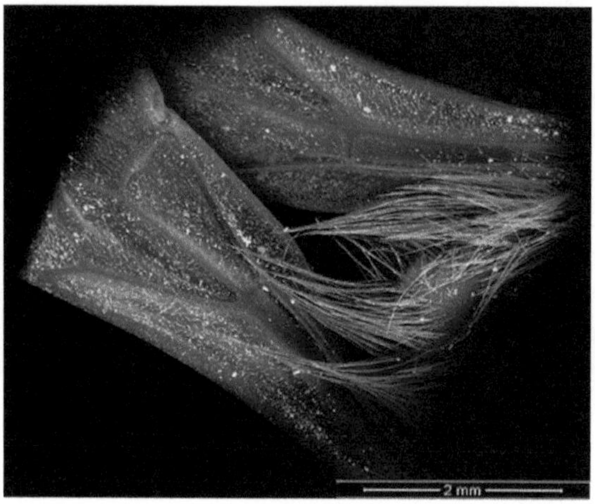

(a)

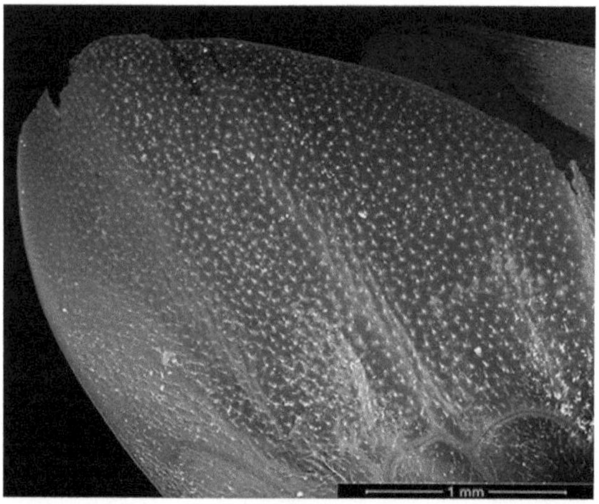

(b)

Figure 3.17 (a) Mouth and (b) wings of a contaminated bumblebee. The greenhouse we set up to study the effects of solid, inorganic and non-biodegradable nanoparticles was divided into two specular sectors, each of which contained the same plants and the same insects (bumblebees). Only one of the two halves of the greenhouse was sprayed with particles. In that part of the greenhouse the bumblebees could no longer fly because of the particles which were deposited on their wings. Because of this, they could no longer feed themselves and they all died. The images show the pollution (white dots) around the mouth and on the wings.

In the course of one of our experiments, we also observed that the particles can settle on the wings of insects, making their flight difficult until it becomes utterly impossible, thereby causing their death. This aspect should be studied carefully and, in any case, taken into consideration when studying the progressive rarefaction of bees, a phenomenon which is probably not only due to the increasing presence of chemical pollutants or the use of pesticides (Fig. 3.17).

3.8 What Is Being Done to Prevent Particles from Entering the Environment?

To be sure, the situation is somewhat curious: We have known all along that breathing and eating dust is bad for our health. Asbestosis, silicosis, bauxite fibrosis, berylliosis, siderosis and byssinosis[a] are just a few among the dust-induced pathologies we have known for many years. Pneumoconiosis, that is, the class of occupational lung diseases caused by the inhalation of dust is a word all doctors know. Nevertheless, we continue to produce finer and finer (i.e. more and more aggressive) dust and allow it to enter relentlessly into the environment, the only one we have available, not yet being able to escape from this planet, if we will ever be. And what is even more curious is that there are 'scientists', luckily enough nowadays a dwindling minority, who still wonder whether particles are really harmful. This for the relief and the joy of industrialists and politicians who, thus, find a 'scientific' excuse to continue undeterred the former to pollute and the latter to allow it.

However, though with some exceptions, the problem is perceived, and the proof is that there are legal and technical systems which, admittedly in a shy and not particularly effective way, try to tackle it.

If, at least in many cases, laws look more like the result of negotiations between polluters and legislators than derived from

---

[a]Byssinosis is an occupational pathology affecting the lungs, caused by cotton fibres. Once we had the chance to be present at a surgical operation on a patient diagnosed as affected by pleural mesothelioma. It was only our electron microscopy observation on the surgical samples that showed that it was not asbestos but cotton to be the cause of the illness.

scientific and medical considerations, technical countermeasures do not seem to be particularly effective either.

This is not a technical book addressed to technicians and engineers, who have much better texts available for their information. So, what little follows is no more than few, simple reflections about a couple of preventive systems currently in use.

At first glance, mechanical filtration could seem the most immediate and reasonable way to stop particles issued from any source.

3.8.1 Bag Filters

Bag filters are very widely used, particularly, though certainly not only, in waste incinerators. They are composed of many long cylinders made of close-woven fabric capable, in the highest-performing products, of resisting a temperature of around 170°C. Through them, dust-laden gas (very often air) is forced, and particles, as happens in the bronchi, are generally captured by four different mechanisms: *inertial collection*, *interception*, *Brownian movement* and *electrostatic forces*. The efficiency claimed, in truth without much explanation, is above 99%, but that numeric datum seems at least questionable. The particles taken into account are only the primary, filterable ones, while the primary condensable and the secondary particles, far more important in terms of quantity, are disregarded. The second questionable point is weight. That 99 point something percent is calculated as the weight of the dust captured. Since, as already mentioned, for simple geometrical reasons, weight is proportional to the cube of the particle's radius; if the filter stops particles whose diameter is 10 μm but can't stop those whose diameter is 0.1 and whose weight is, therefore, one-millionth of the former particles, efficiency, at least at first glance, looks very high. Unfortunately, the smaller the particle, the more penetrating it is, and bag filters are inefficient as regards nanoparticles. So, that claim does not take real efficiency into account with regards to health, missing condensable and secondary particles and, what is even more important not in terms of weight but in terms of health, small-sized ones. It must also be added that, not to clog the filters, what they capture is made to drop to the bottom of the system together with the ash which accounts for roughly 1/3 of the mass of what is being burned in a waste incinerator.

The obvious conclusion, if scientific data and nothing else are considered, is that incineration is a technique by which waste is, at least in part, made to disappear from view (though hidden in various ways, ash does not disappear) but is transformed into something which is far more aggressive for health and environment. Only to be added marginally: each ton of waste needs as much quantity of other material to be treated (water, methane, ammonia, bicarbonate, active carbon, etc.) and all those materials must somehow be disposed of.

3.8.2 Urban Pollution Filters

A few years ago, we had the opportunity to work in New Delhi (India) with an air filtration system similar to what we experimented on the roof of a bus in Rome (Figs. 3.18–3.20). What we tried in India was a device which was not in motion but was placed in a square, much larger in size than the one we used in Rome, where the air entered mechanically sucked and then was emitted purified. Its efficiency was very high, but its range of action was limited, with the aggravating circumstance of having continuously polluted air

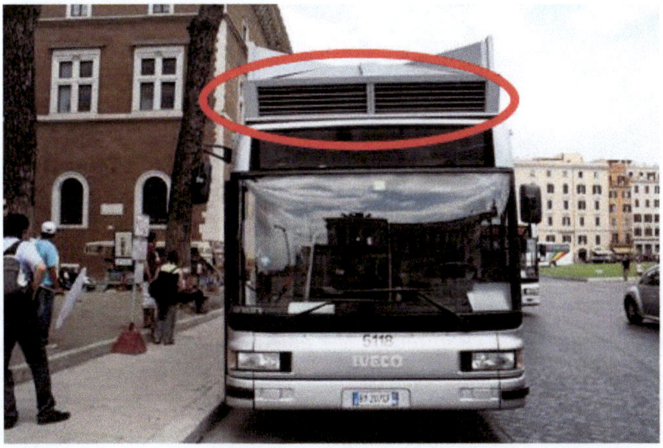

Figure 3.18 Electro-filter system located on the top of a bus in Rome.

arriving. Therefore, such a system would have been excellent in a closed place such as, for example, an airport indoor environment, but in fact it proved to be ineffective outdoors. The particles found show an extremely serious pollution situation with particles also composed of uranium and thorium as well as a large variety of other chemical elements.

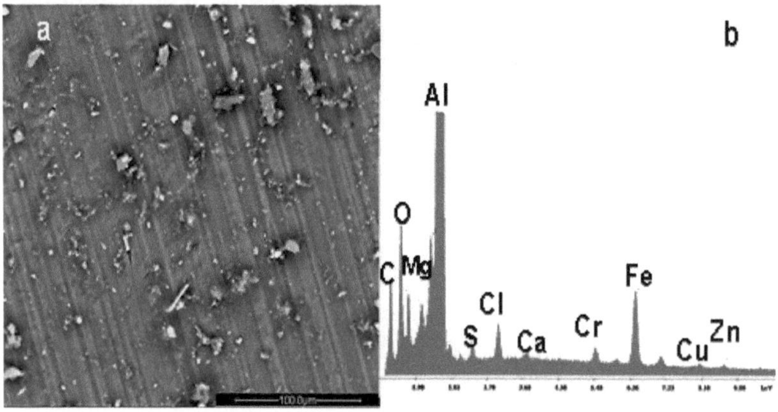

(a)

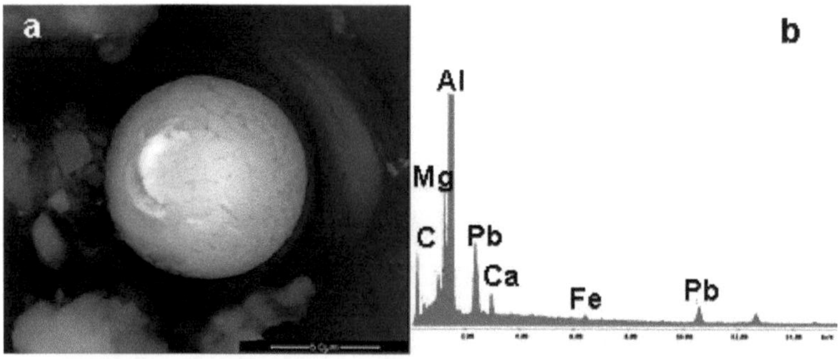

(b)

Figure 3.19 (a) Pollution identified in the electro-filter system in Rome. The particles are those captured by the electro-filter of the filter box placed on the roof of the bus which circulated in Rome for a week. Their shape and composition shows what floats in the air of a big city. (b) The spherical particle shown in the photograph comes from the air of Rome. Its shape demonstrates a high-temperature origin. Many iron-based particles were identified, few of lead.

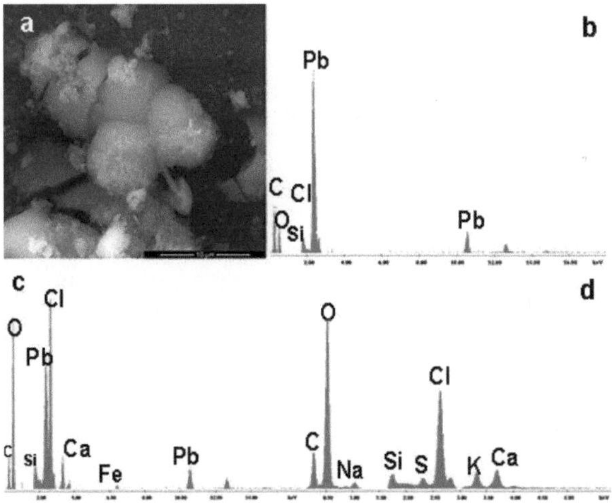

(a)

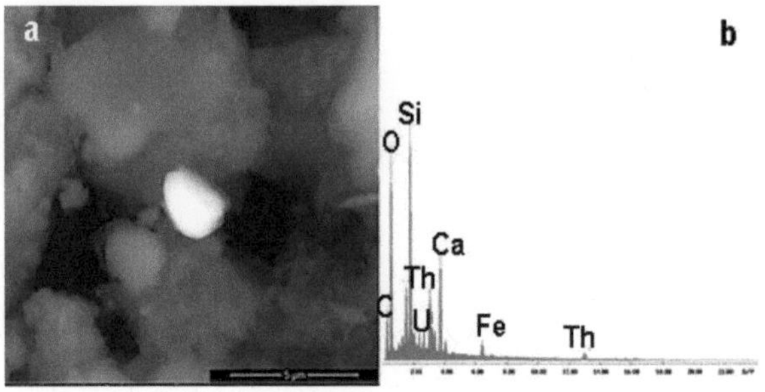

(b)

Figure 3.20 (a) Pollution identified in the static electro-filter in New Delhi, India. The presence of lead-based particulate matter found in New Delhi most likely originates from gasoline which still contains tetraethyl lead as an anti-knock. In countries where that substance has been banned for several decades, the lead pollution it has caused still remains in the environment. (b) A particle containing also uranium and thorium which are radioactive, demonstrates how toxic the pollution we inhale every day is.

References

1. http://www.who.int/ionizing_radiation/pub_meet/en/Depluranium2.pdf.

2. http://www.nrc.gov/docs/ML0322/ML032230109.pdf.
3. Anke, M., Seeber, O., Müller, R., Schäfer, U., and Zerull, J. (2009). Uranium transfer in the food chain from soil to plants, animals and man. *Chemie der Erde – Geochemistry*, **69**, pp. 75–90.
4. http://avalon.law.yale.edu/sept11/epa_002.asp.
5. http://www.asbestos.com/world-trade-center/.
6. http://courses.washington.edu/overney/NME498_Material/NME498_Lectures/Lecture4-Overney-NP-Synthesis.pdf.

Chapter 4

Exposure to Air Pollution: How Particles Enter the Body

The ways through which micro- and nanoparticles are introduced into the body are various, and we have already discussed the topic in several publications, including the already mentioned books *Nanopathology: The Health Impact of Nanoparticles* (Pan Stanford Publishing, now Jenny Stanford Publishing, 2008) and *Case Studies in Nanotoxicology and Particle Toxicology* (Elsevier Academic Press), whose reading is essential for the best understanding of what follows.

4.1 The Inhalation/Respiration Pathway

When particles, particularly the smaller ones, are issued into the atmosphere, no matter how and from what source, their behaviour is, under many aspects, similar to a gas's. Because of their tiny size and mass, they can float suspended in the air and be inhaled. If their size is small enough (typically, though not exclusively, below about 0.5 μm), they can get as deep as the alveoli, the about 600 million hollow structures connected to the bronchioles located at the distal ends of the alveolar ducts. Around them, thin vessels bring venous blood whose content of carbon dioxide diffuses inside the alveolar cavity, while oxygen, arrived in the alveoli through inspiration,

Advances in Nanopathology: From Vaccines to Food
Antonietta Morena Gatti and Stefano Montanari

ISBN 978-981-4877-29-9 (Hardcover), 978-1-003-05622-5 (eBook)
www.jennystanford.com

diffuses out to enrich the arterial blood, which is carried away from the lungs to reach all tissues. Expiration empties the alveoli of carbon dioxide.

Every day we breathe about 11,000 l of air (much more do active athletes), and inevitably, we inhale a huge quantity of particles suspended in the atmosphere. A considerable number of these particles are deposited in the respiratory tract, depending on their size, density, shape, electric charge and surface properties. The breathing pattern and the health state of the lungs of the individual are also of great influence on the phenomenon. Most particles entering the respiratory tract are expelled through expiration. This effect decreases its efficacy as the lungs and bronchi lose their functionality. If an excessive quantity of mucus coats the lower bronchial tracts, as can happen, for instance, in smokers, particles have greater probability to slide towards the cul-de-sac formed by the alveoli. Expulsion is even more problematic when the cilia present in the respiratory tract are shorter or, in any case, less functional or are not functional at all, conditions associated, among others, with tobacco smoking, with cancer or with genetic disorders (e.g. Kartagener syndrome).

Generally speaking, most particles with an aerodynamic diameter[a] less than 10 μm stop in the nose or in the throat and cannot penetrate further in the respiratory tract.

Deposition in the lungs occurs by one of four different ways: *interception*, *impaction*, *sedimentation* and *diffusion*.

- Interception happens when the particle travels so close to a surface of the airway passages that an edge of the particle touches their surface. This kind of deposition is typical of fibres (e.g. asbestos, cotton, etc.). The fibre length is crucial to determine where the particle is going to be intercepted.
- Impaction: When particles travel inside the bronchial system, they do not follow the air when it bends in the airway system but tend to continue along their linear trajectory and impact against the bronchus wall, where they tend to stick. Particle's mass and velocity influence the likelihood of impaction. The higher those two parameters, the higher the likelihood.

[a]Aerodynamic diameter is the diameter of a spherical particle which has the same settling velocity as another particle regardless of its shape, size or density.

- Sedimentation: Gravity and air resistance will eventually exceed particle buoyancy, so particles will settle on an inner surface of the bronchi and the bronchioles. Sedimentation is an important factor with larger particles.
- Nanoparticles tend to diffuse according to the Brownian motion and deposit on the bronchial walls mostly by chance. Diffusion is the prevalent mechanism for deposition in the small airways and alveoli, where only small particulate matter is present.

Once particles are inside the alveoli, they cross their wall in a matter of a few tens of seconds entering the bloodstream. For that reason, they have little or no possibility to induce particular reactions involving the lungs.

In vivo studies of the University of Leuven verified that 100-nm-sized particulate matter, once inhaled, can cross the lung barrier in 60 s and disperse in the blood circulation [1–3]. Within an hour they can reach the liver and the kidneys. The percentage of particles not trapped in these organs can continue to travel throughout the body, reaching all organs, none excluded.

The entrapment can also occur in the upper respiratory tract (mouth, nose, trachea) where a pathology may originate.

The example of the nose cancer (Chapter 3) of the farmer living in the close vicinity of a waste incinerator is just one of many possible examples.

Of course, the particles which don't enter the bloodstream and remain in the lungs can induce a pathology as well. The variety of lung tissue reactions ranges from granulomatosis to fibrosis to cancer. The type of reaction depends essentially on the characteristics of the particulate matter, namely morphology, size, chemical composition and degradation/corrosion. Peritoneal mesothelioma is a typical cancer of the serous membrane which wraps the lungs. The peculiarity of the lung mesothelioma induced by asbestos particulate matter depends on the morphology of the asbestos (a mineral fibre with one dimension at the nanoscale) and on its partial degradability once inside the extracellular fluids.

The following images (Fig. 4.1) give an example of what type of pollution can be found inside the lungs. The lungs collect everything of the environmental/industrial/occupational pollution inhaled, leaving a specific print. Beyond particles of 'normal' pollution (tungsten, antimony, etc.), elements of rare earth are detected like shown in Fig. 4.1.

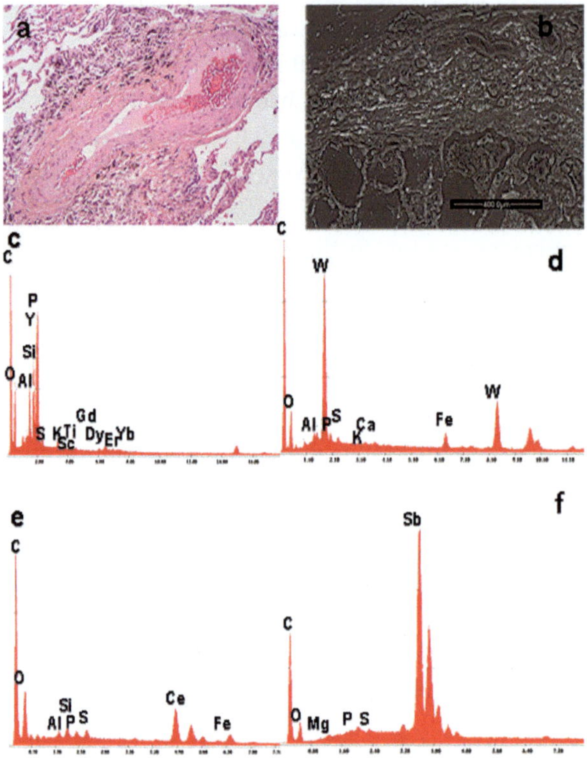

Figure 4.1 Examples of particulate matter entrapped in the lungs. The traditional histological image of optical microscopy of a lung tissue does not give the possibility of accurately identifying the content of solid and inorganic particles. The same tissue observed with the electron microscope shows the particles clearly and makes it possible to determine their elemental chemical composition.

Of particular interest are the studies of Oberdörster et al. showing that inhaled particles can have 'access to the central nervous system and ganglia via translocation along axons and dendrites of neurons' [4].

This observation is particularly important because it could provide fundamental tips for the understanding of diseases such as amyotrophic lateral sclerosis (ALS), also known as Lou Gehrig's disease, or, in any case, for understanding diseases involving a progressive paralysis such as the one we have described on page 142 of the book *Nanopathology: The Health Impact of Nanoparticles* (Pan Stanford Publishing, now Jenny Stanford Publishing, 2008).

A correlation between what had been inhaled and lung cancer was already made, and it is easy to find inside the cancer an important concentration of all the particulate matter inhaled and captured during the patient's life, including urban, industrial and occupational pollution [5].

Recently, the World Health Organization (WHO) released a report [6] describing how every year 7 million deaths are due to the exposure to fine particles present in polluted air which lead to diseases such as stroke, heart failure, lung cancer, chronic obstructive pulmonary diseases and respiratory infections, including pneumonia.

The report only considers cardiopulmonary diseases, while particle pollution can affect virtually any organ.

A case which is rarely considered is that related to the small thrombi which the particles induce in the microcirculation, thus preventing the normal flow of blood to the tissue with all which follows from it.

However, or, at least, in most instances, the particles carried by the bloodstream can reach any organ and tissue, whose general behaviour is very similar to that of any mechanical filter: they capture the particles without, then, as far as we know, being able to get rid of them.

The massive introduction of sub-micron- and nanosized particles in the environment, in food and in drugs increases the exposure of everyone to these stimuli which can interest the whole body. This novel bio-interaction is not yet well described in the books, even if many research projects of nanotoxicity were supported by the European Commission, research organisations and foundations.

Much of what results from the research depends on the cultural background of the researchers, a background which is often refined but equally often too specialised.

Biologists stress the biological aspect, biochemists the biomolecular, histopathologists the morphological, geneticists the DNA and environmentalists focus on particulate matter. As was to be expected, psychiatrists also come into play, according to whom many diseases derive from alterations of the psyche and for this reason are treated with psychotropic drugs. In parentheses, we have had experience of cases treated for years with anxiolytics, anti-depressants, neuroleptics, sedatives, sleeping pills, tranquilizers, etc., because of the alterations in the behaviour of the patient (generally, though not always, a soldier) on which the diagnosis was made, when the problem was a brain tumour which had become intractable due to the loss of time. It is very sad to be right only on the autopsy table.

In any case, all contributions are welcome, and all those specialists, with different techniques, with different magnifications, with different 'eyes' see a portion of the pathological phenomenon.

What is needed is synthesis through a multi-disciplinary approach, which is now largely missing, where everyone must be open and willing to accept that bacteria, viruses, chemicals, particles or psyche exist or matter, where each excludes or minimises the other.

4.2 Particles and the Circulatory System

Once they enter the body through the lungs or the digestive system, particles travel in the blood. There they can interact with red and white blood cells, proteins, enzymes and other blood components. That interaction is regulated by properties like physical adhesiveness, electrostatic forces, chemical affinity, covalent bonds, hydrogen bonds, van der Waals forces, etc. [7].

Resuming what is written in Chapter 1, at the end of the nineties, studying caval filtration (see appendix, Chapter 1), we had already observed that particles can transform fibrinogen, that is, the soluble glycoprotein factor I of the coagulation factors, into fibrin (factor Ia) (see Chapter 2) (Fig. 4.2).

In the majority of subjects, particles are carried by the bloodstream, following its destiny, that is, reaching any organ and tissue. As to particles, it is impossible to predict whether all particles are captured by tissues and organs or, if they are, when. In fact, analysing blood samples, particles can always be found, but we can't tell whether they have just entered the bloodstream or they have been there for a long time.

Our studies on leukaemia and cryoglobulinaemia identified statistically meaningful quantities of micro- and nanosized foreign bodies in the blood of these patients (Figs. 4.3 and 4.4) [3].

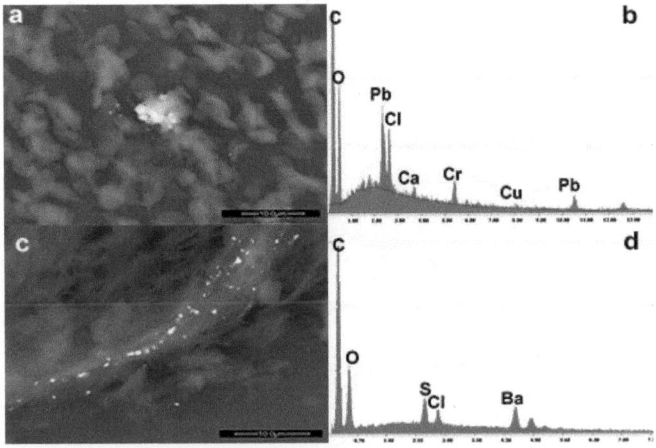

Figure 4.2 Particle identified in a thrombus of a myocardial infarct and fibrin bundle. Ba-S particles (d) had fibrinogen transformed into a fibrin bundle (c) in a thrombus. Pb-Cl-Cr-Ca-Cu (b) particles found in a coronary vessel affected by a myocardial infarct.

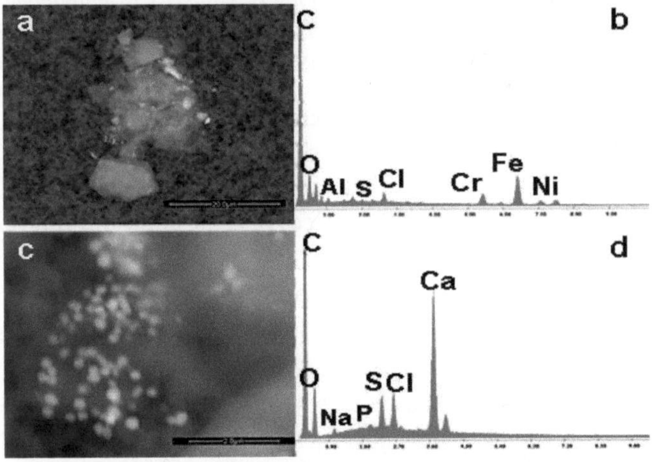

Figure 4.3 Particles in a patient's blood affected by leukaemia. The particles shown in the images have been identified in the blood of a subject with acute myeloid leukaemia. The steel-based particles (iron, chromium and nickel) are obviously of exogenous origin. The presence of relatively coarse particles is worth noting, which, due to their size, cannot have entered through the pulmonary alveoli but, with great probability, by ingestion. The calcium-based particles, on the other hand, are almost certainly of endogenous origin and are characteristic of several forms of cancer.

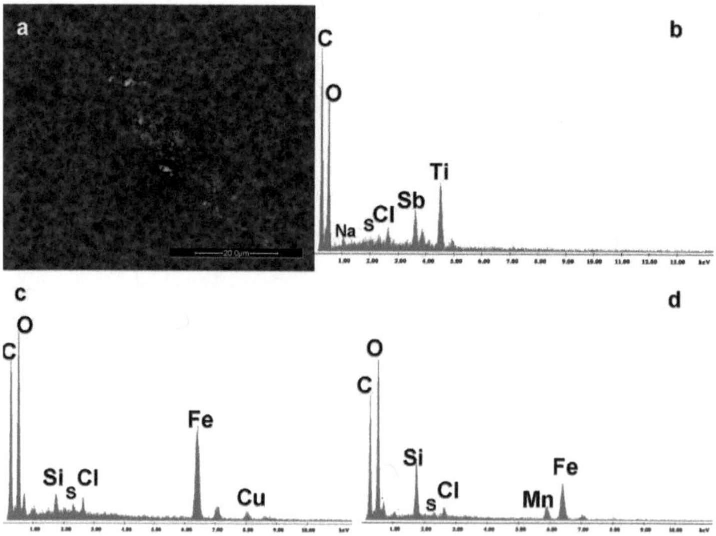

Figure 4.4 Particles in a patient's blood affected by cryoglobulinaemia. Simple (monoclonal) cryoglobulinaemia or type-1 cryoglobulinaemia consists of the presence in the serum of an isotype or sub-class of immunoglobulins (Igs), which precipitate reversibly below 37°C. It is one of many orphan diseases of unknown origin. However, in the cases we have been able to examine, the serum contained, as in this case, numerous non-biocompatible metallic inorganic particles. The patient was affected also by hepatitis C virus.

In both pathologies, leukaemia and cryoglobulinaemia, we found not only foreign bodies but also traces of their nano-bio-interaction.

There is a direct correlation between the presence of internalised foreign bodies and how blood reacts. The type of reaction depends mainly on the particle's size, its morphology, its chemistry, its free energy of surface and its superficial electrical charges.

Particles can also adhere to erythrocytes. When particles are numerous enough, they can cover a significant part of the red blood cells' external surface, thus hindering their ability to carry oxygen and carbon dioxide (Fig. 4.5).

Once, we had a chance to examine a tract of descending aorta affected by an aneurism and found a concentration of particles embedded in the wall, while the healthy portion of the artery was 'clean' (Fig. 4.6).

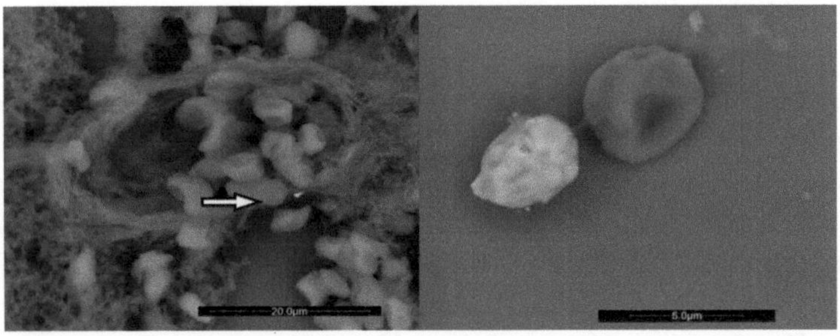

Figure 4.5 Red blood cells with particles. Most of the particles which enter the body are carried by the blood, where they can also interfere with red blood cells. One of the possibilities is to deform them, as can be seen in these photographs.

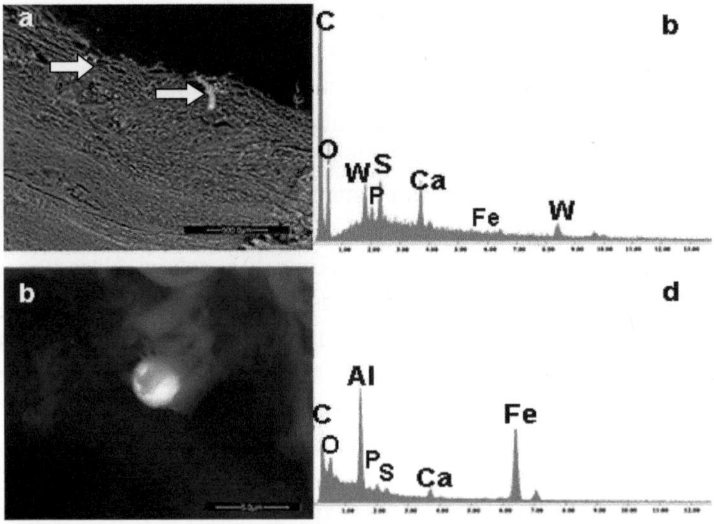

Figure 4.6 Aortic aneurysm. We have no evidence to demonstrate the responsibility of solid and inorganic particles in causing an aortic aneurysm. Our case history includes only one case and, therefore, is completely insufficient to affirm anything. The only thing we can say is that the wall of the aneurysmal aortic tract we analysed contained particles of clear external origin (a spherical particle of just under 3 µm in diameter is shown in a photograph), while the healthy tissue did not contain any particulate pollutants.

Having only one case available, we could not give an explanation to what we were observing, the question being whether the particles had somehow caused the aneurism, perhaps because, being solid and hard, they had scratched the intima, or had been attracted there by the already damaged tissue or the altered hydrodynamics of the blood. In our opinion, the former possibility is less probable, since, for hydrodynamics reasons, the blood flow speed close to the wall is very slow, in fact, close to zero, so the particles would be unlikely to physically harm the intima. It is also hard to believe that those particles could have had the time to exert a biological action on the arterial wall. In any case, the problem requires further research based on an appropriate series.

4.3 The Environment: Polluted Sites

It is a widely known notion that all inhabited areas and, in particular, those with industrial settlements are polluted.

The consequences of pollution are not always immediately visible, and one example among many may be the situation on the southeast coast of Australia devastated by fires between the end of 2019 and the beginning of 2020. Regardless of the serious ecological problems caused by the loss of such vast expanses of vegetation, the ashes will inevitably cause negative consequences on flora and fauna, starting from those of microscopic dimensions. Already a few weeks after the fires occurred, the ashes fallen into the water had caused the death of a large number of fish, but the particles are not unlikely to also interfere with the DNA. Therefore, the consequences will become clearly visible only over the years.

Some examples of these contaminations were studied is in a research project of nano-ecotoxicity called INESE by the Italian Institute of Technology of Italy [9–13].

In Chapter 3 we have already discussed the generation of a new pollution due to war and terrorism. The exposure of humans and animals to these new contaminants can be the cause of new symptoms and new pathologies, not infrequently in the form of syndromes, that is, of sets of different symptoms, many of which are not described or barely mentioned in medical texts because of their novelty.

By now, there are highly polluted territories all over the planet and, in fact, impossible to reclaim.

An example may be that of the so-called 'Terra dei Fuochi' (Land of Fires), a vast territory which extends over an area hard to circumscribe accurately between the Italian provinces of Naples and Caserta. In that area, industrial residues and waste of largely unknown quantity and nature coming not only from Italy are poured in every day for decades. In addition, huge quantities of waste are continually set on fire. As often happens almost everywhere, the problem has been long ignored and, in the same way, frequent cases of cancer, miscarriages and foetal malformations of humans and animals have been underestimated or ignored at all. Now, as was obviously to be expected, the pollutants have infiltrated the soil to an unknown depth and, in any case, a depth which probably varies from site to site, depending on the quantity and type of waste and the quality of the soil. Local aquifers have certainly not been spared.

Now, belatedly, money is being allocated to reclaim those territories. What has been done in certain circumstances is to dig a few metres deep in limited areas and move that soil to places where people are unaware of what they are receiving.

In fact, recovering those territories is impossible. As for aquifers, beyond more or less questionable techniques, it is essential to realise that rainwater which almost always enters the underlying aquifer passes through polluted soil, dragging pollutants with it.

Most people believe that there is always a solution for any problem, but unfortunately, this is not the case.

4.4 The Aerotoxic Syndrome

Nanopathology is a novel concept, a possible key to understanding new pathologies, new syndromes, such as the so-called aerotoxic syndrome, a set of symptoms which affect airline crews and sometimes even some passengers. The epiphenomenon which indicates the occurrence of the toxic event is what is described by those who participated in it as a smell of wet dog or dirty socks. Then, a light and not always visible cloud is released inside the aircraft cabin. Such an occurrence is known as 'fume event' (Fig. 4.7) [15, 16].

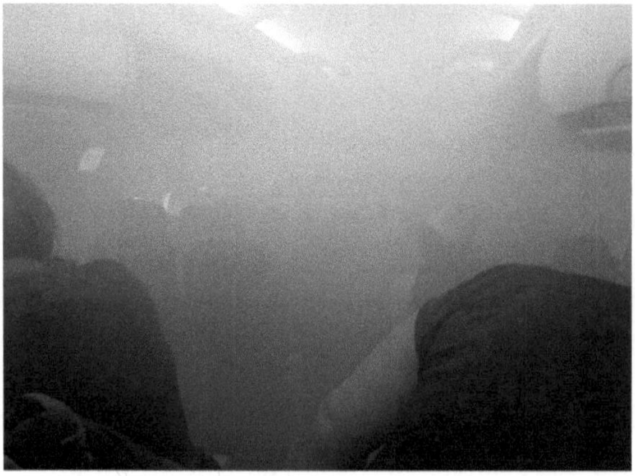

Figure 4.7 Fume event in an aircraft. The image shows the effect of a fume event inside an aircraft. A sort of smog is dispersed in the aircraft cabin. Figure courtesy of the Aerotoxic Association.

When these conditions occur, the crew may be no longer able to reason properly and carry out normal activities, which, as is evident, is particularly critical with regards to the pilots.

In these cases, emergency landings are used. In others, fortunately rare, accidents occur which remain officially unexplained.

Among a number of possible examples, on 25 October 2016, an accident happened to the British Airways A380 flying from San Francisco to London, which was diverted to Vancouver in an emergency, where 25 people, the crew and some passengers, were taken to the hospital for the umpteenth case of 'fume event'.

In those events, immediately after landing, the crew and, in some cases, the passengers are transported to the hospital and generally discharged after short hospitalisations.

The symptoms they declare are confusion, balance difficulty, severe headache, cognitive difficulties and emotional changes (great restlessness and aggression), and skin irritation (particularly in the face and arms).

The problem becomes more and more serious for the cabin crew, who, unlike passengers whose exposure is only occasional, can suffer the phenomenon with a certain frequency. Thus, to the symptoms listed above, others are added: severe hair loss, insomnia, swollen eyes, poor eyesight with photophobia, extreme fatigue, slight hearing loss, palpitations, fluctuating blood pressure, muscle weakness with severe pain, sciatic pain, stiff neck, alcohol intolerance and fragrance intolerance – a set of symptoms which is partially similar to that of a multiple chemical sensitivity.

Unfortunately, unlike what rarely happens with other pathologies, thanks to homeostasis, these symptoms tend to worsen over time, so much so that the crew, less and less able to tolerate the environment inside the plane, quit the job, and some crew members whose cases we dealt with have become completely unable to lead a normal life.

In the silence of both media and airlines, some pilots reported that their colleagues died from the aggravation of the symptoms. Nothing is known, however, of intoxicated passengers. It is possible that, having been victims only once of the event, they recovered perfectly as it is equally possible that their symptoms remained or even worsened without the doctors to whom they turned being able to find an explanation.

Without going into technical details which do not fall within our competences and the purposes of this book, an explanation of the phenomenon which, however one wants to deal with it, is real and repeats itself, despite attempts to minimise its scope, it must be considered that the air which is introduced into the cockpit of some models of aircraft passes through the engines, where it is compressed and heated [16].

For a number of reasons (malfunctioning, wear, age, etc.), that air may contain organic and inorganic pollutants coming from the lubricant: carbon monoxide and carbonaceous combusted particles, hydrogen cyanide, hydrogen fluoride, hydrogen chloride, nitrogen oxide, sulphur dioxide, ammonia, acrolein and combusted tricresylphoshate [17, 18]. As in the case of internal combustion engines in automobiles, also in this case solid and inorganic particles are formed by combustion.

At this point, it is necessary to take again into consideration a concept as basic as too often overlooked of toxicology: one plus one does not equal two. When two toxic substances are present together, except in rare cases, the sum of their toxicities is higher than that which would be obtained with a simple arithmetic addition of the two effects. When, as is the case we are dealing with, there are many pollutants involved, their combined effect is almost impossible to predict. What is certain is that it is much higher than what one might suppose by evaluating the substances

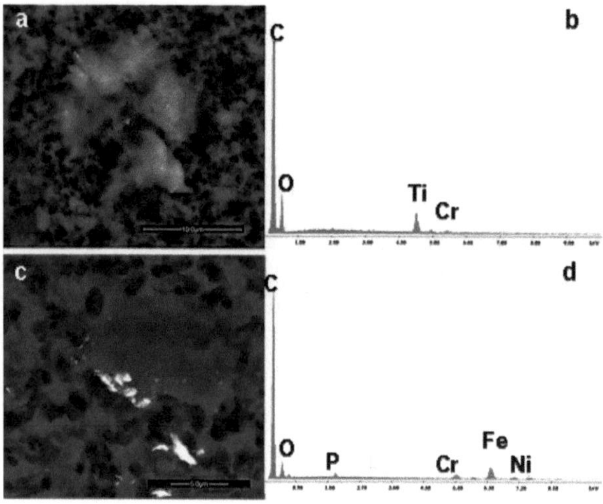

(a)

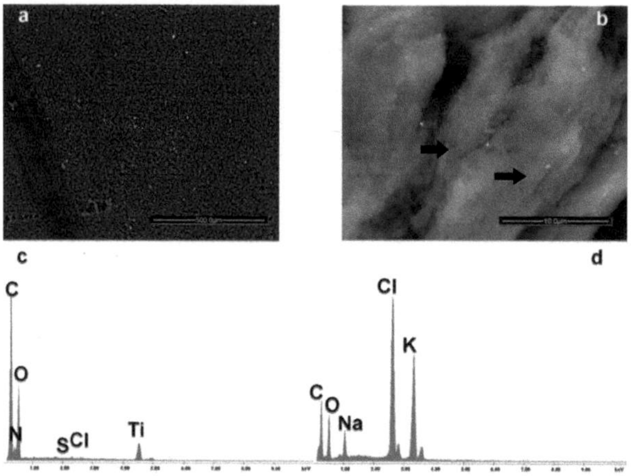

(b)

Figure 4.8 (a) Examples of pollution inside the oil to lubricate the engine. The particles shown in the photograph were identified in the lubricating oil of the engine. (b) Examples of particles dispersed in the aircraft. The particles are those captured by a filter placed at the entrance of the air into the cockpit environment of an airline. The compressed and heated air comes from the engines and is breathed by crew and passengers. Titanium and iron come from mechanical wear, while carbon, chlorine, potassium, sodium and sulphur come from pyrolysed oil.

individually. The problem is aggravated when the exposures are repeated, given the fact that those substances can accumulate in the body and can trigger states of sensitisation, even very serious ones. In view of this obviousness, minimisation attempts look naive to say the least, and the attempt to impose silence is the most certain means of not solving this like any other problem.

Not too rarely, what is put in place is the attitude of the majority of companies. So, if one faces the problem from a purely immediate economic and temporally limited point of view, it is understandable that after the fume event has occurred, the interior of the aircraft is not thoroughly cleaned, the oil is not changed and no overhaul is made of the air acquisition, treatment and delivery systems, including with this also the engines (Fig. 4.8).

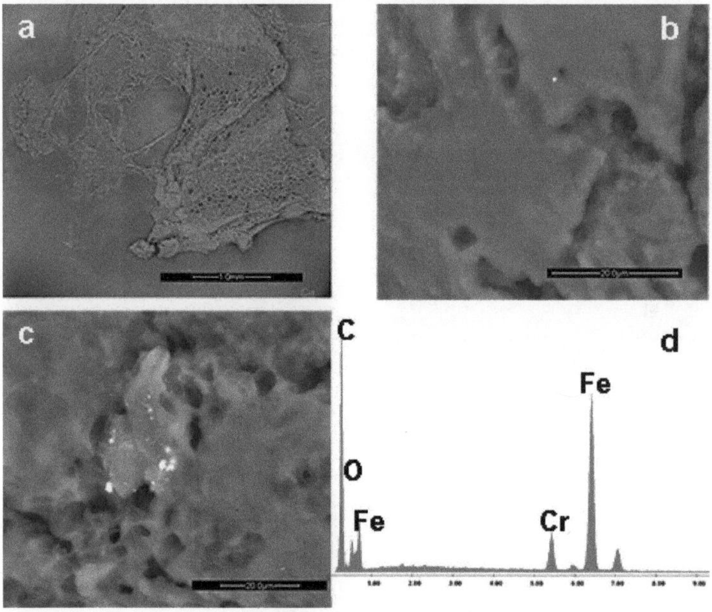

Figure 4.9 Diseased pilot's fatty tissue. The particulate matter seen in the photographs was contained in the fatty tissue of an airplane pilot who had been forced to quit his job due to repeated exposure to smoke events. Similar particles, mainly composed of steel as they are, can probably come from the air introduced inside the cabin of the aircraft after passing through the engines. The particles seized in the fat can be released into the blood in the case of weight loss.

The hypothesis we conceived and which, free from understandable vested interests, seems reasonable to us is that the pathology is due to the inhalation of a mixture of gases, organic molecules and particulate dust composed of an inorganic core coated with organic compounds. So, the acute symptoms can be due to the mutual interaction of all toxic compounds in the blood circulation and in the brain, while the chronic symptoms can be due to the long-term presence of the inorganic ones in the organs and tissues, including also fat. Fat can be of particular importance because, when it is consumed (and the fact is particularly visible in cases of rapid weight loss), the particles it contains are released within the organism to reach other tissues and organs.

We had the possibility to analyse some biological samples we got from ill patients or from their families if the patient had already died. The following images (Figs. 4.9 and 4.10) show part of these biological findings.

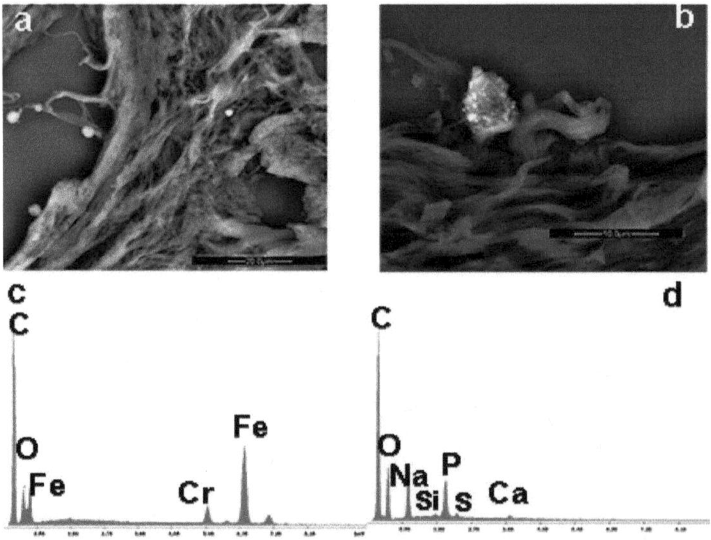

Figure 4.10 Dead pilot's brain. The particles shown in the images were detected in the brain of a deceased airplane pilot who suffered a series of fume events. The steel is most likely derived from the passage of the air which is introduced into the cabin of the aircraft after passing through the engines. Phosphorus-containing particles are likely to originate from the lubricant used in those engines.

4.5 Diffusion and Concentration of Particles

As we have already briefly described, the particulate pollutants we deal with can remain suspended in the atmosphere for a very long time. When they finally touch the ground, a little wind is enough to lift them up again and restart the journey. In addition, as repeatedly stressed, most of the solid and inorganic particles are not degradable, and therefore, the journeys they make due to physical diffusion phenomena, wind, changes in atmospheric pressure, Coriolis fictitious force, rain, etc., can last for a very long time, covering long distances, thus allowing a sort of homogenisation at a planetary level. It must be taken into account that polluting particles can have very different sizes, from a few nanometres of aerodynamic diameter up to tens of microns, with all that this entails in terms of mass and, therefore, in terms of the time during which they can remain for a more or less long time suspended and move.

Another necessary consideration is to remember that particles can either crumble, as is the case with the fragile, spherical and hollow ones, or aggregate with each other and, as is characteristic of secondary particulate matter, stick with non-particulate chemical substances such as dioxins and furans more or less occasionally present in the atmosphere. In addition to the consequence of becoming a carrier of organic pollutants which would not otherwise have a great chance of travelling, joining necessarily means increasing mass and volume with all which follows. On the other hand, as is obvious, crumbling means giving origin to more numerous and lower-mass particles.

Because of all this, the diffusion patterns of the polluting particles currently applied are often oversimplifications with significant margins of error.

If one considers a polluting source, it is evident that the concentration of the particles is especially high in its vicinity and decreases with distance. For this reason, the quality and quantity of particulate pollutants appear different from area to area and, in some way, characterise it. The images of cities suffocated by pollution are known to everybody, and it is equally well known that we always rely on atmospheric events to mitigate the situation.

Given the fact, it must be added that part of the fallen particles seriously affects the composition of the soil up to the aquifers by changing their characteristics; this too must be taken into account when assessing the impact of a polluting source on a certain territory. It is usual that when bureaucratic permission is required to install a plant which emits pollutants, documentation is presented which refers exclusively to that particular plant as if it were the only source of pollution in the area and on the basis of that documentation the permit to be built and to go into operation is released. Almost never the authorities in charge take into consideration how that particular pollution adds to what is already present and, perhaps, to pollution coming from areas which are not close. Again, the toxicological concept that one plus one equals a higher sum than two is valid.

In the course of our investigations on the environment, we dealt with relatively large polluting sources such as heavy-oil power plants, waste incinerators, foundries and cement factories. Each of them has profoundly affected more or less vast expanses of territory.

Each source of pollution has its own peculiarities, and micro- and nanoparticles are excellent markers which can be found both in samples taken from the environment and in patients' tissues. And it is not rare that it is from the analyses on the particles contained in pathological tissues that it is possible to trace the source of pollution. In several cases, such scientifically irrefutable evidence has been used in criminal courts.

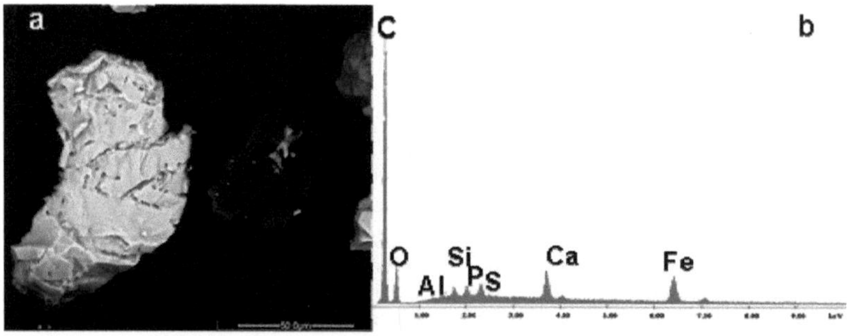

Figure 4.11 Cast iron industry pollution. The so-called 'Ferriera di Servola' is an industrial complex dating back to 1896 specialised in the production of cast iron, located in a district of the Italian city of Trieste, in an area now quite densely inhabited. From its smokestacks, fumes containing generally coarse iron-based particles come out and fall into the surrounding area. Significant quantities of dust can be collected daily anywhere in the vicinity.

The following images (Figs. 4.11–4.14) witness the dispersion of the industrial pollution in the surrounding environment of factories.

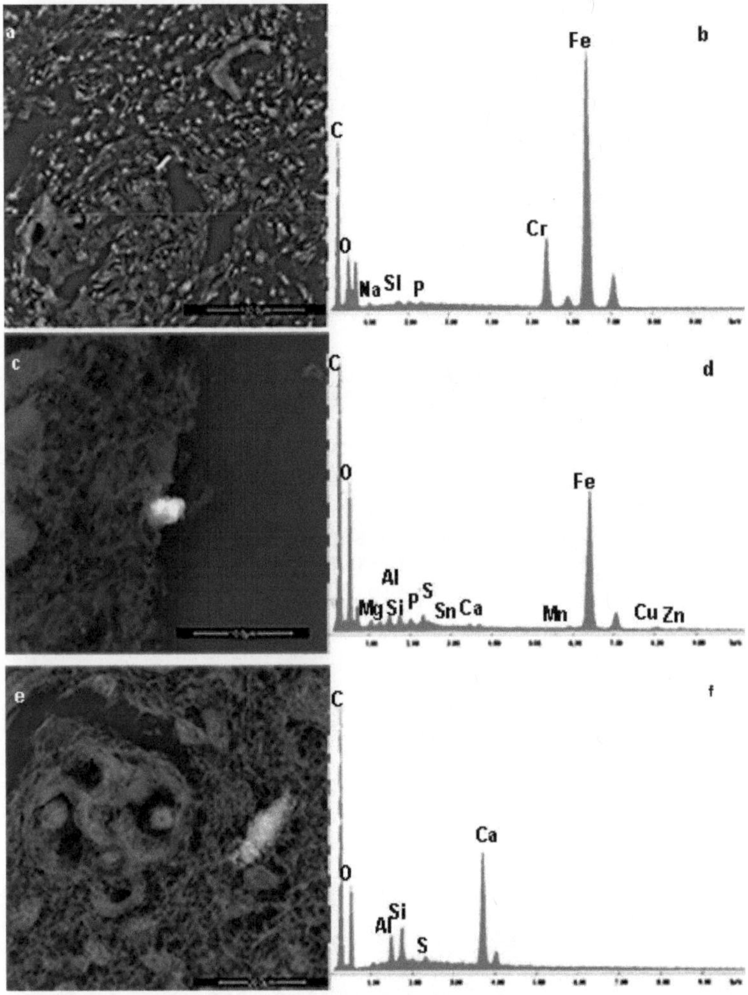

Figure 4.12 Steelwork pollution in a child's brain. The particles shown in the electron microscopy images were detected in the brain of a child who died of brain cancer at the age of 5. The boy lived in the Italian town of Taranto, where one of the largest foundries in Europe has stood for decades. The ferrous particles are typical of the pollution of that territory, while those based on calcium probably formed inside the cancerous tissue, as is quite characteristic of those pathological conditions.

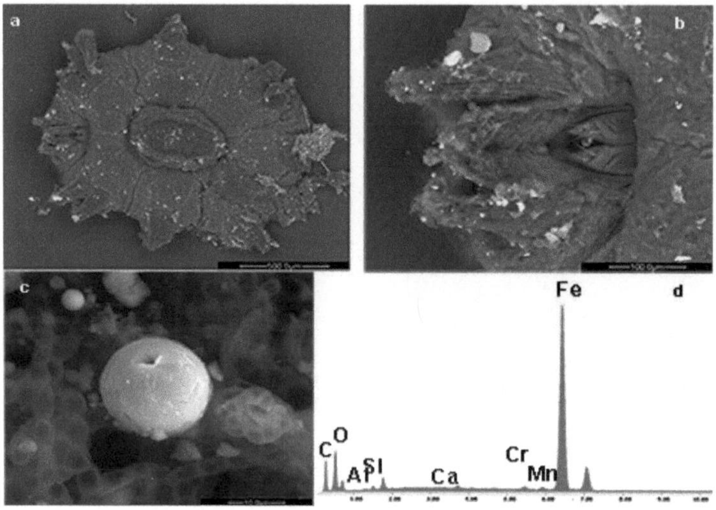

Figure 4.13 Steelwork pollution in an insect. Some samples taken in the air, on leaves, on metal objects and on windowsills in an area around a large foundry located in the industrial area of Udine (Italy) showed the obvious presence of spherical particles typical of the castings. That type of pollution which had existed for many years had damaged the small orchards and the gardens around the houses. Among the exhibits, we also collected a dying insect sprinkled with particles, as can be seen in the two low-magnification photographs.

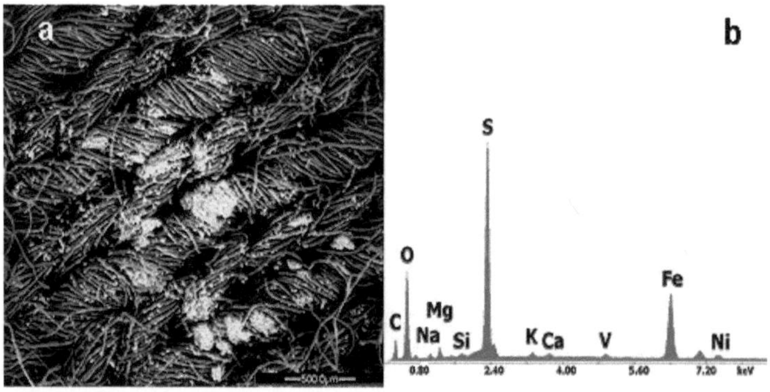

Figure 4.14 Heavy-oil power plant pollution on a T-shirt. Inside the Italian river Po Delta Regional Park, there is a power plant once operating with heavy oils, which has been inactive for a few years. The fallout from the fumes polluted a relatively vast, once uncontaminated area. The particles were so aggressive that they corroded the bodywork of cars. The particles shown in the photographs were contained in oily droplets fallen on a T-shirt hanging out to dry. The local criminal court instructed us to determine whether the fallout with

(Continued)

which the inhabitants of the area complained actually came from the thermal power plant. The presence of vanadium, an element which is not often found in polluting particles, was constantly detected both in the fuel used by the plant and in the particles found in the numerous finds examined. This, together with other tests, analyses and evidence, allowed us to establish with certainty the origin of the fallout.

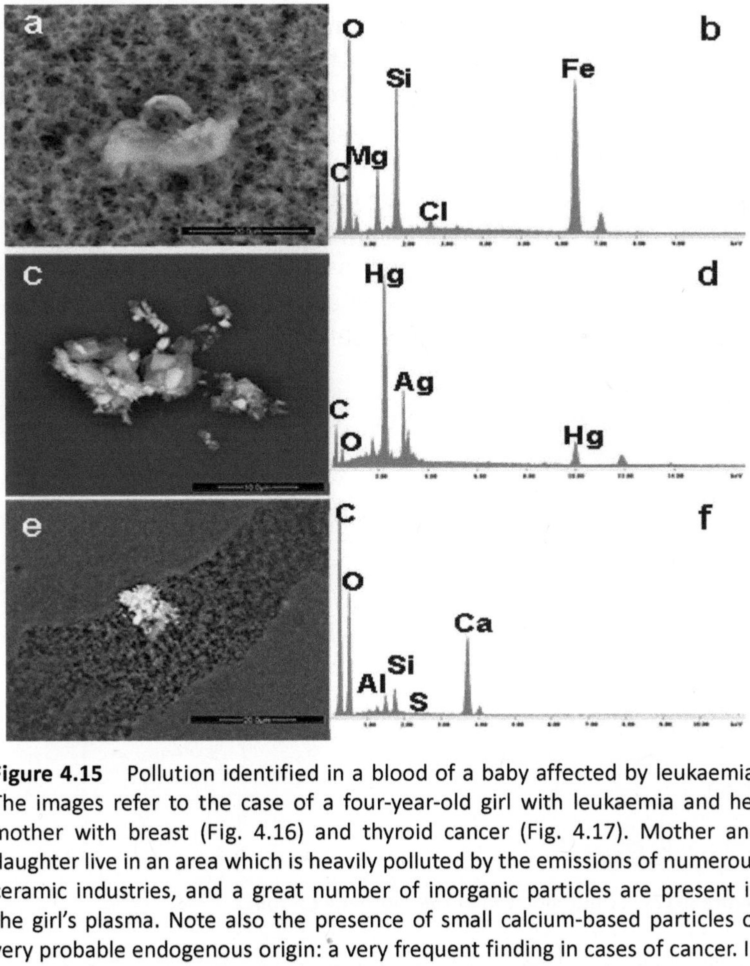

Figure 4.15 Pollution identified in a blood of a baby affected by leukaemia. The images refer to the case of a four-year-old girl with leukaemia and her mother with breast (Fig. 4.16) and thyroid cancer (Fig. 4.17). Mother and daughter live in an area which is heavily polluted by the emissions of numerous ceramic industries, and a great number of inorganic particles are present in the girl's plasma. Note also the presence of small calcium-based particles of very probable endogenous origin: a very frequent finding in cases of cancer. In both breast and thyroid biopsies of the mother, the presence of solid, inorganic particles is evident. Again, the cancerous tissues contained small calcium-based particles. It may be interesting to note the greater complexity from the point of view of the elemental chemical composition of the particles present in the thyroid compared to those of the breast.

One of the cases we came across is that of a four-year-old girl with leukaemia (Fig. 4.15). In the area where the family lives, there are many industries which produce ceramic material, almost exclusively tiles. The little patient's mother had worked for some time in one of those industries and had suffered from breast cancer. She has recently been diagnosed with thyroid cancer (Figs. 4.16 and 4.17). It is interesting to note that particles of an origin ascribable to the ceramic industries are present in the girl's blood and in the mother's biopsy samples. It should be added that what is emitted from the chimneys of those industries is quite varied, because, in addition to the basic materials, glazes, dyes and different chemical products are used, which can be different from company to company. To this pollution is added that of the very intense traffic of trucks used for the transport of raw materials and finished products.

It would have been interesting to have been able to analyse the cerebrospinal fluid which was taken every week from the child, but unfortunately, the doctor in charge refused to give us a sample.

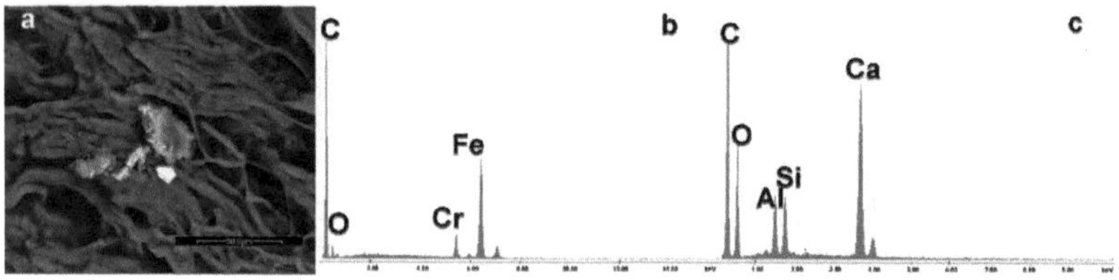

Figure 4.16 Contamination identified in the breast cancer of the mother.

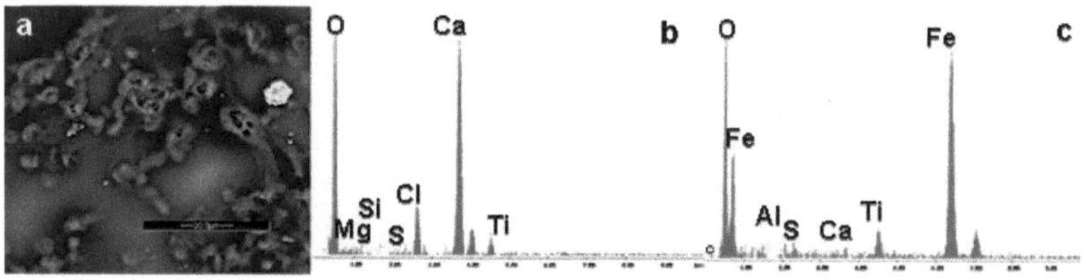

Figure 4.17 Contamination of the mother's thyroid.

References

1. Nemmar, A., Hoylaerts, M. F., Hoet, P. H., Vermylen, J., and Nemery, B. (2003). Size effect of intratracheally instilled particles on pulmonary

inflammation and vascular trombosis. *Toxicol.Appl.Pharmacol.*, **186**(1), pp. 38–45, https://doi.org/10.1016/S0041-008X(02)00024-8.

2. Nemmar, A., Hoet, P. H., Vanquickenborne, B., Dinsdale, D., Thomeer, M., Hoylaerts, M. F., Vanbilloen, H., Mortelmans, L., and Nemery, B. (2002). Passage of inhaled particles in to the blood circulation in humans. *Circulation*, **105**(4), pp. 411–414, https://doi.org/10.1164/rccm.200602-301OC.
3. Visani, G., Manti, A., Valentini, L., Canonico, B., Loscocco, F., Isidori, A., Gabucci, E., Gobbi, P., Montanari, S., Rocchi, M., Papa, S., and Gatti, A. *(2016)*. Environmental nanoparticles are significantly over-expressed in acute myeloid leukemia. *Leuk. Res.*, **50**, pp. 50–56, http://www.sciencedirect.com/science/article/pii/S0145212616301916.
4. Oberdörster, G., Oberdörster, E., and Oberdörster, J. (2005). Nanotoxicology: an emerging discipline evolving from studies of ultrafine particles. *Environ. Health Perspect.*, **113**(7), pp. 823–839.
5. Hamra, G. B., Guha, N., Cohen, A., Laden, F., Raaschou-Nielsen, O., Samet, J. M., Vineis, P., Forastiere, F., Saldiva, P., Yorifuji, T., and Loomis, D. (2014). Outdoor particulate matter exposure and lung cancer: a systematic review and meta-analysis. *Environ. Health Perspect.*, **122**(9), pp. 906–911.
6. https://www.who.int/airpollution/data/en/.
7. Gatti, A. (2016). Nano-biointeraction and nanopathology. *News Medical Life Sciences*, http://www.news-medical.net/news/20161031/Nano-biointeraction-andnanopathology.aspx.
8. Gatti, A. and Montanari, S. (2015). *Case studies in Nanotoxicology and Particle Toxicology*. Elsevier, London, p. 260.
9. Gambardella, C., Ferrando, S., Gatti, A. M., Cataldi, E., Ramoino, P., Aluigi, M. G., Faimali, M., Diaspro, A., and Falugi, C. (2015). Morpho-functional and biochemical markers of stress in sea urchin life stages exposed to engineered nanoparticles. *Environ. Toxicol.*, **5**, doi:10.1002/tox.22159.
10. Vittori, L., Carbone, S., Gatti, A., Vianello, G., and Nannipieri, P. (2015). Uptake and translocation of metals and nutrients in tomato grown in soil polluted with metal oxide (CeO_2, Fe_3O_4, SnO_2, TiO_2) or metallic (Ag, Co, Ni) engineered nanoparticles. *Environ. Sci. Pollut. Res.*, **22**(3), 1841–1853, https://www.researchgate.net/publication/265394076_Article.
11. Vittori, L., Gatti, A., et al. (2015). Impact of cobalt and silver nanoparticles and ions on soil microbial community structure, lumbricusrubellus

health and their trophic interactions. *Environ. Toxicol. Chem. BiolFertil Soils*, **51**, pp. 261– 269.

12. Gambardella, C., Ferrando, S., Gatti, A., Cataldi, E., Ramoino, P., Aluigi, M. G., Faimali, M., Diaspro, A., and Falugi, C. (2016). Review: Morphofunctional and biochemical markers of stress in sea urchin life stages exposed to engineered nanoparticles. *Environ. Toxicol.*, **31**(11), pp. 1552–1562.
13. Vittori Antisari, L., Carbone, S., Bosi, S., Gatti, A., and Dinelli, G. (2018). Engineered nanoparticles effects in soil-plant system: basil (Ocimumbasilicum L.) study case. *Appl. Soil Ecol.*, **123**(2), pp. 551–560.
14. https://www.paddleyourownkanoo.com/2019/10/06/yet-another-fume-event-on-a-british-airways-flight-brings-total-to-56-in-less-than-months/.
15. https://www.thelondoneconomic.com/lifestyle/health/testimonies-of-devastating-cost-to-public-health-of-toxic-passenger-jets-submitted-to-the-hague/18/10/.
16. https://787updates.newairplane.com/getmedia/0a6b6209-6b19-4dce-9afb-81ba391102de/Cabin-Air-Contaminants-Boeing-backgrounder.
17. Winder, C. (2006). Hazardous chemicals in jet aircraft: case study-jet engine oils and aerotoxic syndrome. *Curr. Top. Toxicol.*, **3**, pp. 65–88.
18. Vyvyan Howard, C., Johnson, D. W., Morton, J., Michaelis, S., Supplee, D., and Burdon, J. (2018). Is a cumulative exposure to a background aerosol of nanoparticles part of the causal mechanism of aerotoxic syndrome? *Nanomed. Nanosci. Res.*, https://www.gavinpublishers.com/articles/Review-Article/Nanomedicine-and-Nanoscience-Research/Is-a-Cumulative-Exposure-to-a-Background-Aerosol-of-Nanoparticles-Part-of-the-Causal-Mechanism-of-Aerotoxic-Syndrome.

Chapter 5

The Ingestion Pathway

5.1 Introduction

As already mentioned, particles float in the atmosphere and are carried mostly by the wind. The smaller their mass, the longer their stay in the air, and the farther they can travel. In the long run, however, they all fall to the ground, and their fall can take place on fruits, vegetables and cereals, where they become part not only of our food but also of that of the animals destined to become our food and of their products. So, those particles are ingested, but most of the times we don't notice.

With an increasing frequency, micro- and nanoparticles are deliberately added to food, drugs and even chewing gums, toothpaste and accessories like toothbrushes and interdental floss, that is, something which is not food but which enters the mouth. Food industries add other inorganic material to the organic food in order to increase some properties (conservation, nutritional, aesthetic, or just commercial purposes). But there is the possibility of another contamination coming from the industrial processes of the food preparation, and that comes by using tools which can release something in the food.

In any case, pollutants and additives are regularly ingested by mostly unaware people. From the qualitative point of view, the biological effects induced by those particles are in no way different

Advances in Nanopathology: From Vaccines to Food
Antonietta Morena Gatti and Stefano Montanari

ISBN 978-981-4877-29-9 (Hardcover), 978-1-003-05622-5 (eBook)
www.jennystanford.com

from the environmental pollution's ones, the only visible difference when observed through an electron microscope being the shape and composition consistency of engineered particles as compared to those produced as a random side effect by sources like, for instance, waste incinerators.

The vast majority of those ingested particles are eliminated mixed with faeces, but part of them touch the walls of the stomach or of the intestines and stay there long enough to be captured by the tissue and, eventually, negotiate it.

The main difference between ingested and inhaled particles is size. While only the finer particles can overcome the barriers of the upper respiratory tract and then those of the progressive narrowing of the bronchial diameter, ingestion offers a much wider passage. So, particles of virtually any size can be found in all the digestive system, and some of them, even as big as a few tens of microns, can be detected in the stomach's and the intestine's wall thickness. Part of them, especially those with a smaller size which are not stopped and kept in the digestive system's walls, enter the bloodstream, like the ones coming from the lungs. Inflammatory conditions, no matter how originated, make the intestine wall particularly permeable to the passage of particles, triggering a vicious circle: particles cause inflammation, and inflammation opens the way to larger and larger particles with a stronger and stronger inflammatory effect.

'Der Mensh ist was er isst', which, translated into English, is 'Man is what he eats.' The sentence belongs to Ludwig Feuerbach and, nowadays as when it was written, keeps being largely misunderstood. Actually, the nineteenth-century German philosopher did not mean anything having to do with food science, but if we take those words in their unintended sense, we can find a lot of truth in them. Man depends on food much more than is generally believed, since food is not a simple fuel for our engine meant to give it the energy necessary to keep our organism alive but is an extremely refined mixture of treasure and poison.

'One-third of what we eat serves to keep us alive. Two-thirds, to keep doctors alive.' The sentence sounds like an aphorism just written but, in fact, can be read in an ancient Egyptian papyrus. From that, we can draw many conclusions, the first of which is that, in the millennia passed since, we have not made great progress.

This book, and, more in particular, this chapter, are not intended as a text of dietetics, and what will be discussed in its pages is only the more or less deliberately planned and more or less known content of particles in what we eat. Some brief mention of other pollutants will be given because, as everything concerning toxicology and as has been said more than once in these pages, poisons do not just add up arithmetically their actions but often those deleterious actions are mutually synergistic, and their results may be totally unexpected.

We said that particles fall everywhere, including vegetables. It is only obvious that, at least in most cases, what is found on the surface of those vegetables can be easily enough washed away, but the particular conformation of certain products does not allow the operation to be successful. Broccoli and cauliflowers, for example, have a very rough surface in whose recesses dust creeps and it is practically impossible to get rid of it, no matter how carefully we wash them. Many cereals such as wheat are ground without having been previously washed, and dust becomes inevitably part of the flour. In addition, flour is rather often polluted by the particles produced by grinding operations and, in particular, by the wear of the machinery used. As a personal experience, we found grain polluted by waste, as it was illegally transported in trucks which, in their previous trip, had contained urban and industrial debris: an operation repeated innumerable times (Figs. 5.1 and 5.2).

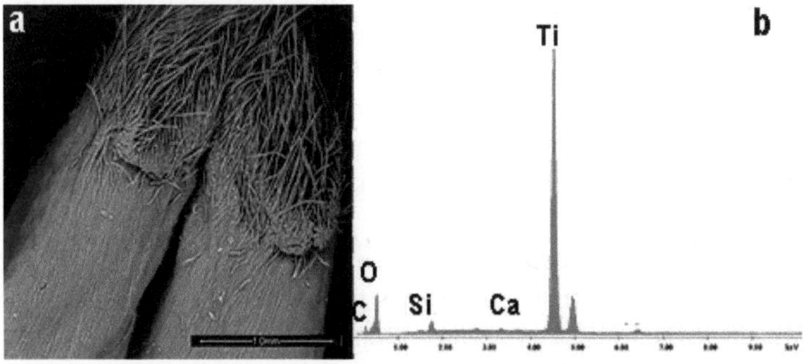

Figure 5.1 Polluted corn. The particles which can be seen in the low-magnification electron microscopy image were attached to the grain kernels recovered from a truck which, before transporting grain, had transported waste of unknown origin. The presence of titanium could only be explained by knowing what the truck had transported before.

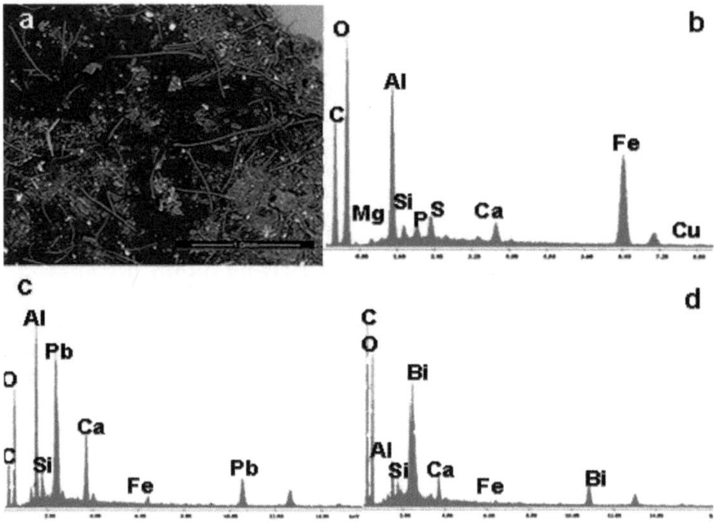

Figure 5.2 Pollution detected in a truck carrying corn. In the truck transporting grain after transporting waste, micro- and nanosized particles with the most varied compositions were detected. Not knowing the type of waste, it is impossible to establish what their origin was. Given the composition, it is not unlikely that at least part of the load was made of incinerator ash. Although it is forbidden to use a truck to transport waste and food, the practice is quite widespread.

But particles fall also on the soil, thus interfering with the growth of plants, and as a matter of fact, this kind of pollution makes organic food, at least as seen from this point of view and disregarding the rest, not particularly different from non-organic, since there is no way to protect crops. Paradoxically, at least if the point of view is only that of the pollutants fallen from the sky, the plants grown in a greenhouse are cleaner and, therefore, healthier than those grown outdoor.

Particles – for example, silver, it being a component of some pesticides – can also be found in fodder for livestock, and that pollutant ends up in their tissues, that is, finally, their meat.

In many cases, fallen or purposely administered particles alter the microflora and microfauna of the soil by changing its chemical characteristics (e.g. through corrosion and the introduction of foreign chemical elements), including pH. This causes the implementation of a selection of the microorganisms to the detriment of the balance necessary for the conservation of the crops.

It must be added that, sooner or later, particles and chemical elements reach the groundwater, a phenomenon which can reach an imposing size below certain landfills. It is important to realise that, as a matter of fact and as already mentioned, purifying an aquifer is technically impossible. One can only stop immediately to pollute and wait for the water contained in the groundwater to be replaced by another which is clean. The phenomenon can take decades but only if the landfill responsible for pollution disappears. Otherwise, the pollution can remain virtually forever.

Non even oceans, lakes and rivers are saved. In addition to the falling dust and directly discharged urban and industrial waste, water contains huge quantities of particles arriving through rivers, and, therefore, even of very distant origin. Unfortunately, those particles, along with other pollutants, can be found in the fish and clams we eat.

5.2 Vegetables

Once we had a chance to analyse an organic cabbage which proved to be polluted by fine basalt dust. The area where that vegetable had been grown was situated on the slopes of Mount Etna (Italy), a volcano which was erupting at the time of collection, so people like us living more than a 1000 km away could ingest those pollutants by eating that cabbage.

Similar events can very frequently happen with flour, a commodity which is often imported from far away, and in most circumstances the buyer does not know anything about the conditions under which the wheat had been cultivated. So, bread, pasta, cookies, cakes and all other flour products can carry a pollution which is unsuspected.

In a study we published in 2009, we showed the results obtained by analysing flour-based foods taken from different countries and continents. In 40% of cases we found them polluted by inorganic micro- and nanoparticles.

The pollution of the flour could have come from various, different sources: from environmental situations where the cereal had grown, from polluted soil or from processing residues, often caused by mechanical metal organs which are worn and whose residues inevitably end up in the flour [1].

Since the flour is imported from countries which can be very far from those where it is processed, it happens to find products polluted by particles which can come from far countries, even from different continents.

One of the current uses of vegetables, not rarely mixed with waste, is as (lignocellulosic) biomasses to be either burned directly in order to generate energy, or to be fermented, thus producing a mixture of gases (carbon monoxide and dioxide, nitrogen oxides, volatile organic compounds whose composition depends on what takes part in the reaction, etc.) which is used as fuel under the name of 'biogas'. The residue of direct combustion is a mix of different ashes which can be used as an additive for fertilizers (in spite of its content of heavy metals, polycyclic aromatic hydrocarbons, chlorobenzenes and other pollutants), while the solid and slurry residue of fermentation called compost is often used as an improver for the quality of soil. The collection we made of plants of chamomile, dandelion and ears of corn in an area over which compost had been spread showed how those vegetables were severely malformed (Fig. 5.3).

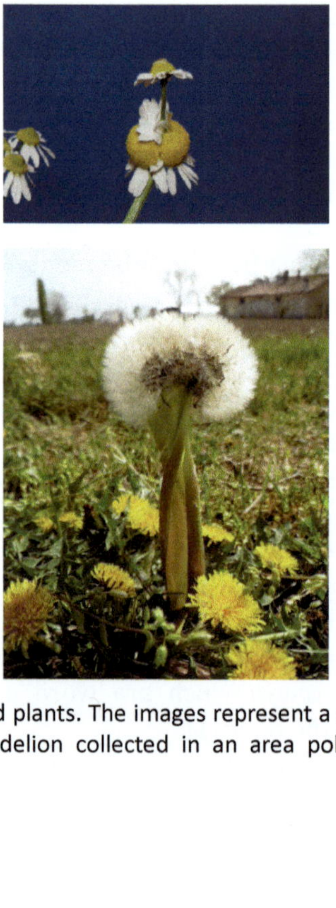

Figure 5.3 Malformed plants. The images represent a malformed chamomile and a malformed dandelion collected in an area polluted by biogas plant compost.

Under the 16th European Biosolid & Organic Resources Conferences (Leeds, UK 14–16 November 2011) a seminar was held, entitled 'Botulism and Other Scares: How Do We Reassure the Public on the Safety of Recycled Organic Wastes'. In that circumstance, Professor Henge Böhnel of the University of Göttingen (Germany) reported that *Clostridium* spores responsible, inter alia, for botulism and tetanus are present in the territories treated with that kind of compost.

There are cases where vegetables currently used as food are polluted on purpose with particulate matter. Polished rice treated with paraffin and then dusted with talc is an example. It should be recalled that talc, when ingested, is a carcinogen to the stomach and that one of its pollutants is asbestos and another is uranium (Fig. 5.4) [2].

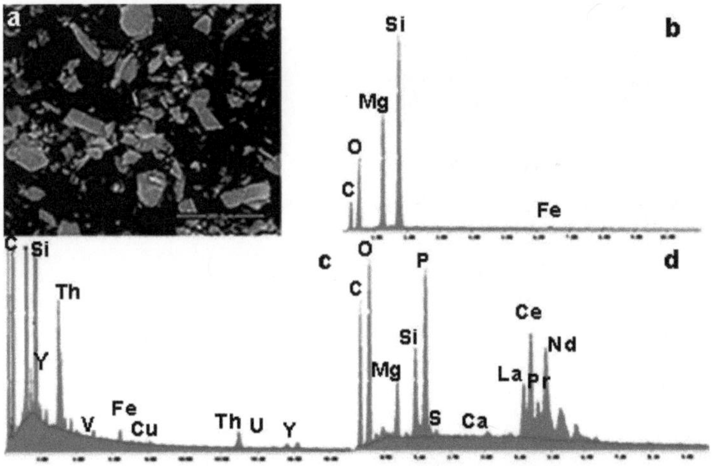

Figure 5.4 Talc. It is a common practice to sprinkle talcum powder on children, especially after washing them. Talc also enters several adult health products. Talc is a mineral reduced to very fine dust down to the size of nanoparticles. Like any other powder, talc can also be easily inhaled and breathed and, as it is not biodegradable, is a potential cause of nanopathologies. The analysis we carried out shows that talc contains thorium and uranium as well as elements such as lanthanum, praseodymium, cerium and neodymium.

5.3 Meat and Fish

Animal physiology is very similar, not too rarely actually identical, to that of humans. So, when animals eat something containing solid, non-biodegradable particles, as already illustrated, part of them are captured by organs and tissues without any possibility to exit. The inevitable consequence is that, when those animals become our food, they introduce those pollutants into our body.

Silver is used as a pesticide, and silver particles can be found on hay and other vegetables used as animal feed. Because of that, detecting them in meat is no surprise at all. But what may be somewhat more worrisome, other particulate matter can also be found in homogenised baby food (Fig. 5.5).

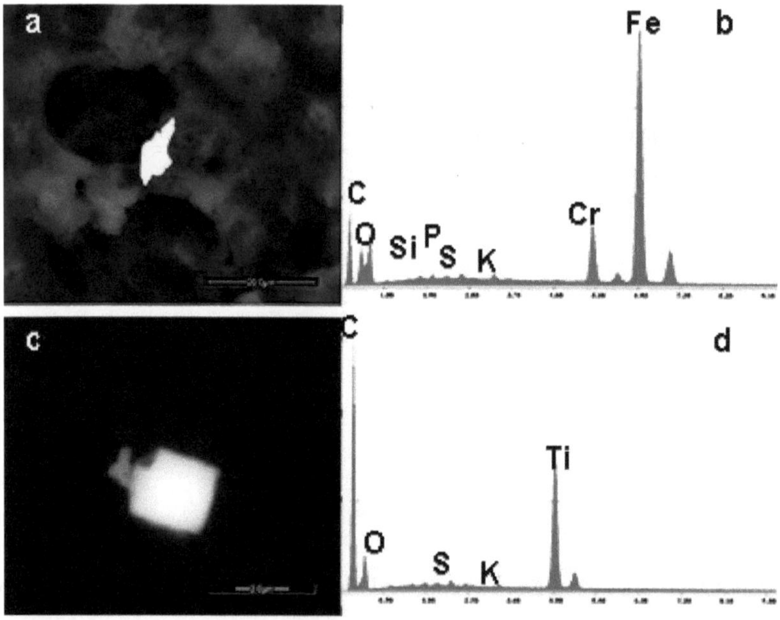

Figure 5.5 Baby food. As is the case with many other meat-based food products, baby homogenised food can also contain solid and inorganic particles. Their origin can be identified both in the raw material (i.e., in the meat and in the residues which the mincing process leaves). In the images shown, the presence of a cubic titanium particle is rather unusual, the sample we analysed being a product of an important brand, and it is clear that controls are not carried out even from official sources which should guarantee safety.

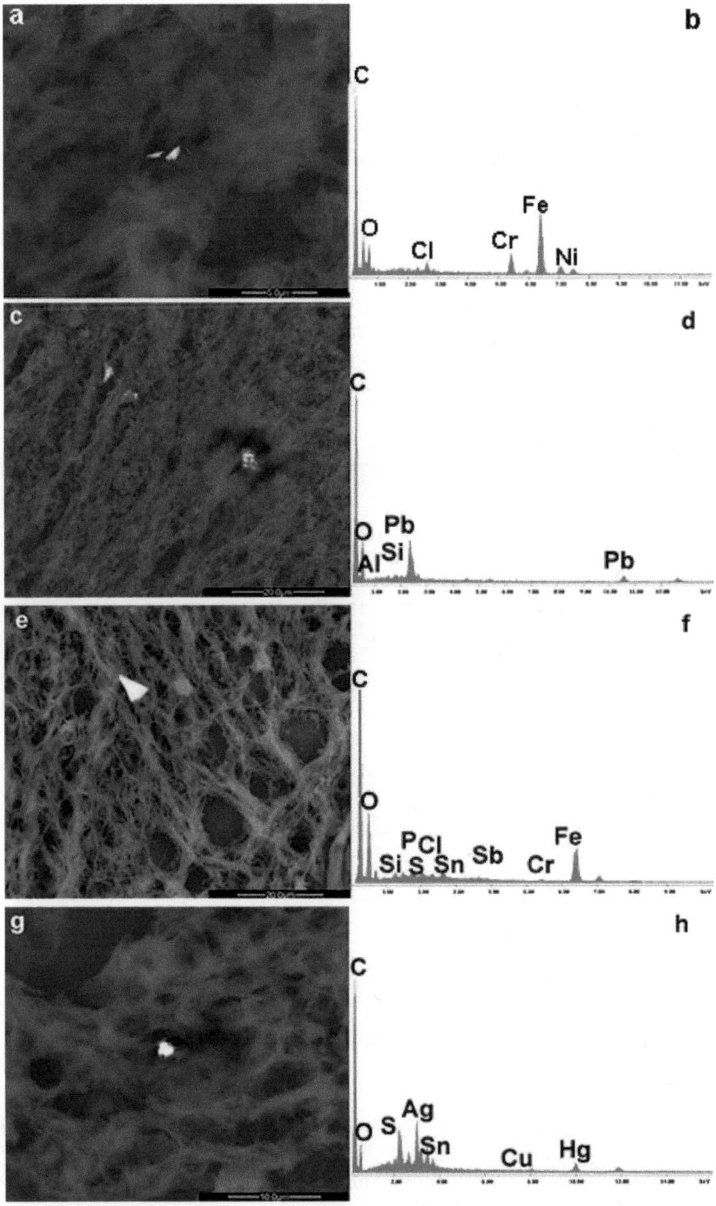

Figure 5.6 Mad cow brain. The analysis of different samples of mortadella, a very common sausage both in Italy and worldwide (where in many circumstances is known under other names), showed how that meat contains steel microparticles.

Quite illegally, there are circumstances in which the flour or the animal meal with which cattle were fed was mixed with exhaust motor oils in order to form a blend and a bolus which could be swallowed without chocking. That oil contains particles coming either from its additives or from the friction between piston and cylinder. Therefore, those pollutants were thus introduced into the animal's organism, including the brain, where they caused serious disturbances to the nerve transmission which works on an electrical basis.

The micro- and nanoparticles in the photographs (Fig. 5.6) belong to the brain of a cow which was ill with bovine spongiform encephalopathy (BSE). The steel-based particles (iron-chromium-nickel) have as a probable origin the residues of the rubbing of mechanical parts of engines lubricated with the used oil which was then added to the feed. The other particles could come from both lubricant additives and from the corpses of other animals transformed into feed.

The reason of that presence is due to processing. To be finely chopped, meat should be frozen, and the processing is performed with blades which quickly lose their sharpness. This involves the loss of residues of the metal the blades are made of and metal particles enter the mixture of minced meat (Fig. 5.7).

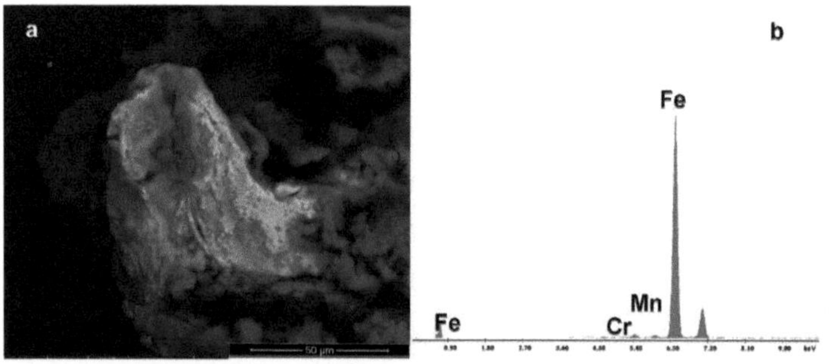

Figure 5.7 Italian sausage. The large particle was photographed in a sample of mortadella, the Italian sausage known abroad under different names. The presence of these metallic residues is due to the wear of the blades with which the frozen meat is minced.

Fish, too, are far from being exempt from particulate pollution. Mercury is the most universally known among the poisons present in fish, particularly big-sized predatory fish like tuna, and the so-called Minamata disease is a tragic example of what that metal, in that case as methylmercury released by a chemical factory, accumulated for decades in the fish and shellfish eaten by the local population. It must be remembered that pollution by particles is different from that caused by atoms or molecules, and when particles, molecules and atoms are present together, it is difficult or utterly impossible to predict the result in terms of toxicity (Fig. 5.8).

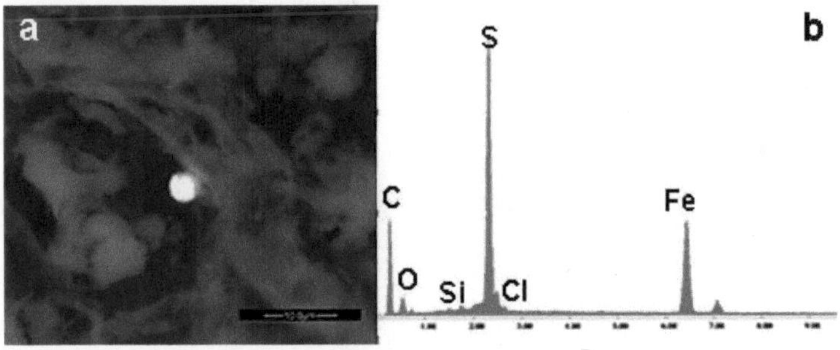

Figure 5.8 Anchovy sample. An increasing quantity of waste ends up in the sea, often coming from rivers and, therefore, from areas which can be geographically distant from the sea. A part of this waste is in the form of micro- and nanoparticles which are excellent markers for pollution because they enter the fish tissue without undergoing transformations as it can happen for many organic substances. In this case, these are iron-based particles which, as evidenced by the spherical shape, come from combustion. The fish analysed was an anchovy.

Technically speaking, foraminifera are members of a phylum or class of amoeboid protists most of which are marine. One of their characteristics is the production of a shell (a 'test') in which they live made of calcium carbonate or agglutinated sediment particles. Like many other very simple beings, foraminifera can represent the base of the food chain (or, better, the food pyramid), and for that reason, they are particularly important, because, if the base is altered, the whole structure is affected in a negative way. When foraminifera live in polluted water, they are malformed with serious difficulties to reproduce. Incidentally, the carbon of the shell comes from the CO_2 dissolved in the water in equilibrium with that present in the atmosphere according to Henry's law. Hence the function of air 'scrubbers' of foraminifera (Fig. 5.9).

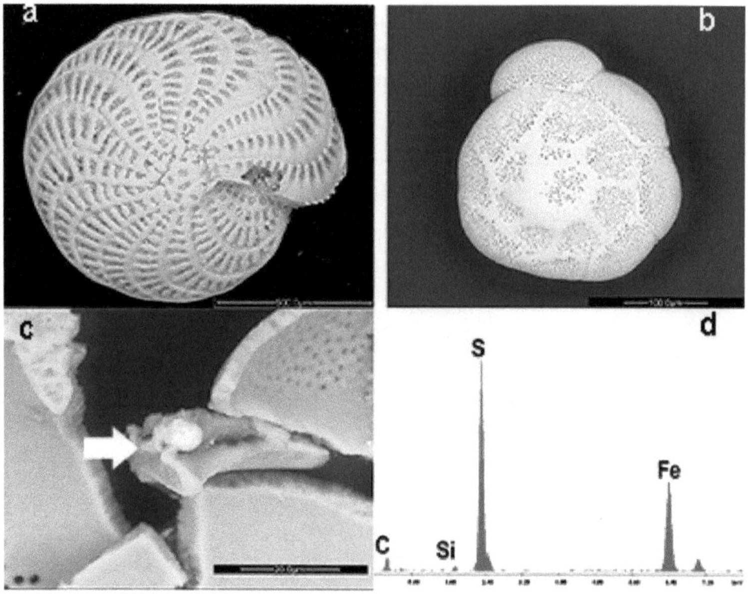

Figure 5.9 Healthy and contaminated foraminifera. (a) A healthy foraminifer, (b) a malformed foraminifer and (c) a polluting, spherical particle (white arrow) which is composed of sulphur and iron.

Particles, especially secondary ones, are the carriers of a number of organic pollutants. Most of them are soluble in fats, and for that reason, they can be found in meat, milk and its derivatives, and eggs. It is important to note that many of those pollutants have a half-life of several years and, as a consequence, remain for a long time in the organism. As already mentioned, part of them, for example, dioxins, are eliminated more quickly by nursing mothers through the milk babies are fed with. Needless to say, the infant will necessarily be exposed to the toxicity of those substances.

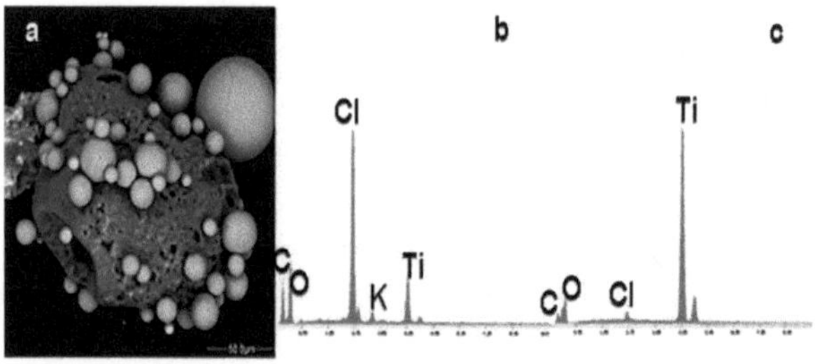

Figure 5.10 Pollution from sparkling candles.

Sparklers are small fireworks emitting sparks, mounted on chopsticks which are used very often, especially by children, on the occasion of parties, and it is also customary to stick them on cakes. To obtain sparks, it is essential to include metals in the composition, each of which gives a different effect. The titanium which we detected in the spark fragments in the case we analysed serves to give the sparks a rich white colour (Fig. 5.10). As it is obvious, those very small metal fragments are inhaled and, if the sparkler is used on a cake, are ingested.

Decorating food, especially sweets, with coloured powders is a very common practice. The image is about a powder sold as gold, but in reality, there is no trace of that metal (Fig. 5.11). The particles, almost all of a rather coarse size, are made up of silicon, aluminium, titanium, potassium and iron. It can be assumed that most of these particles are eliminated in the faeces, but it is also necessary to consider how the gastrointestinal walls allow the passage to much larger particles than it is for those which pass through the respiratory system. It should also be added that it is not at all improbable that these indigestible particles, like titania shown in Fig. 5.12, exert an inflammatory action, thereby making the walls even more permeable.

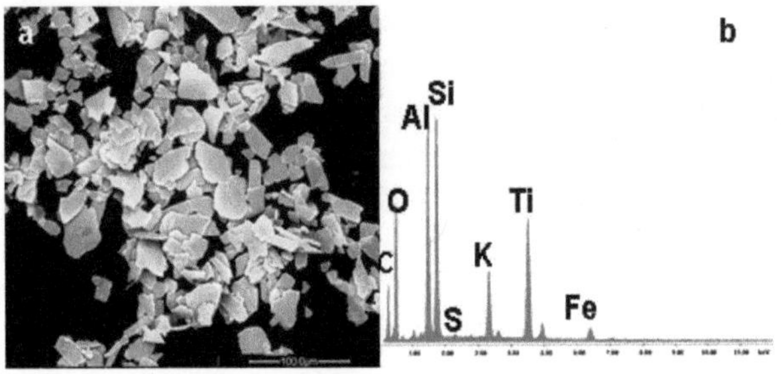

Figure 5.11 'Gold' for cake design.

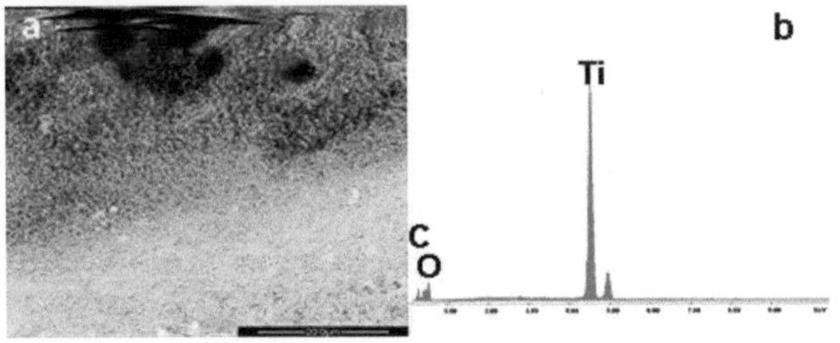

Figure 5.12 Titanium dioxide (titania) nanoparticles to make white icing for cake design.

5.4 Engineered Particles in the Food

As already mentioned, nanoparticles behave in a way which is often different from that of the same material at the macroscale, and with increasing frequency, industry takes advantage of those characteristics. They are used as colouring (e.g. candy coating) and thickening agents in processed food (e.g. mayonnaise), and there are fruits, for example, bananas, which are coated with engineered nanoparticles to retard their spoilage. Nanoparticles are used to purify water (e.g. silver), as anti-caking, clarifiers and gelatin-forming agents (e.g. alumino-silicates) and in packaging to protect food against UV light and prevent the growth of microbes or detect microbial contamination.

As to silver, nanoparticles are now widely used in domestic equipment to filter drinking water in order to avoid bacterial contamination, for packaging, in toothbrushes and in toothpaste, deodorants, medical bandage, etc.

They are also incorporated in polymer-based packaging from which they can be released into food in concentrations increasing according to storage duration. Silver nanoparticles with diameters of 22, 42, 71 and 323 nm were fed to mice at 1 mg/kg over a 14-day period. A size-dependent distribution pattern was found among different organs. The particles smaller than 100 nm were detected in the brain, liver, kidneys and testes, while the largest particles were not seen there. The amount of silver discovered in the brain, lungs and testes was roughly inverse to the particle size [3].

As to alumino-silicate clays, it is known for a long time that they can perturb normal nutrition via their sequestration of minerals and possibly other nutrients. The effect is beneficial to animals which occasionally ingest them to be able to gain nutritional benefit from food which contains toxins, but very little is known about chronic effects on the human organism.

Titanium dioxide is probably the material most nanoparticles added to food are made of, and it is hard to tell how much of it we ingest daily. Those particles are not soluble in water and have three natural forms: rutile, anatase and brookite. Rutile and anatase particles are used to produce pigment-grade material for the colouring of some foods and may be coated with various materials (aluminium, silicon or polymers) to enhance their technological properties. Those coatings are made because they modify the reactions between the surface of the titanium dioxide particles and the matrix where they are mixed, resulting in lower aggregation and a better dispersion possibility (Fig. 5.13).

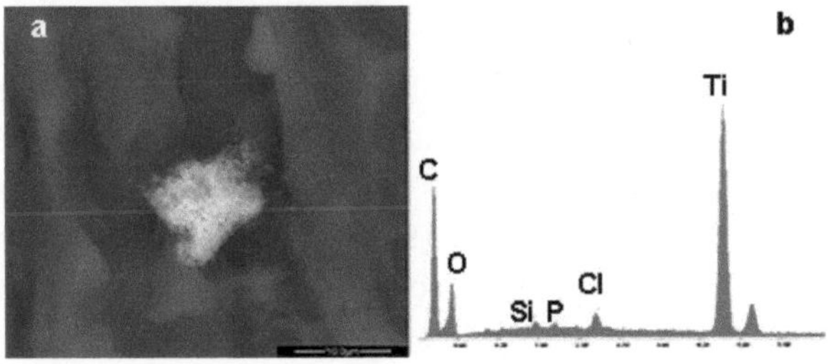

Figure 5.13 Cluster of titania nanoparticles found in a stomach cancer patient.

Nanoparticles are also used in food supplements as addition of iron and trace elements. Their bio-availability, however, is, to say the least, very doubtful. Bio-availability, defined here as the rate and extent to which a component of a food can be used by the organism, varies from individual to individual and, in the same subject, depends on his/her occasional state of health. In any case, many inorganic, insoluble particles cannot be degraded and stored or immediately made available to metabolism. So, the element listed in the label is actually there but, at least in some circumstances, is useless when not harmful at all.

Unfortunately, the current international rules do not distinguish clearly between particles and the same material in bulk. Therefore, when the quantitative limits for inorganic pollutants exist, they are considered on materials whose size and, consequently, whose behaviour is utterly different from its micro- and, more in particular, nanoform. Until this truism is entered in the concepts used by legislators, not only will the confusion remain, but we will be in a constant state of legally ignored risk. The immediate consequence is the use of nanoparticles in an increasing number of products, unfortunately including food.

The attitude of producers towards nanoparticles is rather contradictory, probably depending on the market approach which the manufacturer (or the distributor) intends to give to the product. There are instances where a content of nanoparticles is reported in the label and nanoparticles are actually there. In other circumstances, instead, no nano, though attested by the producer, but larger particles are present (it should be remembered that nanoparticles have a great tendency to agglomerate). Yet, in other cases, the chemistry declared is not the one detected by the analysis as is the case of gold or silver, declared by the manufacturer but in fact not always present. And, finally, there are nanoparticles which are actually contained in the product, but no notice is given. For some time, there are marketed products labelled as particle-free as a proof that people grow more and more suspicious towards nanoparticles and that neither lawmakers nor producers have managed to make the least clarity in this regard. As has often happened in other circumstances, even science looks uncertain, but it must be considered that the vast majority of what is done in terms of research is financially supported by industry. The consequences are the doubt and the actual possibility, as history teaches us, of biased results, great confusion in data interpretation and delays in official and universally accepted understanding of facts which, objectively, do not seem to leave room for conflicting interpretations.

Not only ingredients but also how food is prepared can be critical. Non-stick containers used to cook food are growing more and more popular. Their inside surface is coated with polytetrafluoroethylene, perfluorooctanoic acid or similar matrices. No matter what they are made of, in those matrices, mineral micro- and nanoparticles are often dispersed, giving an attractively shiny appearance to the pot or pan. All the containers we tested in our laboratory showed that those particles come off easily, going to pollute the food, even if the surface looks intact (Fig. 5.14).

Strictly speaking, chewing gum is not a food, but is often used the same way as a confectionery such as candies. In some types of those products, solid micro- and nanoparticles with an abrasive function are added. The chewing movement will partially clean the teeth from food debris, but many particles are ingested by swallowing saliva.

As previously mentioned, there are no reasonable laws, not to mention controls, ruling, even if only for the sake of prudence, the use and the presence of particles. As a matter of fact, in this way, manufacturers are free to act as they want, adding particles (be they micro or nano) either boasting their presence or being silent about it, while consumers remain without reliable information, without the possibility to choose among a great variety of products and without protection.

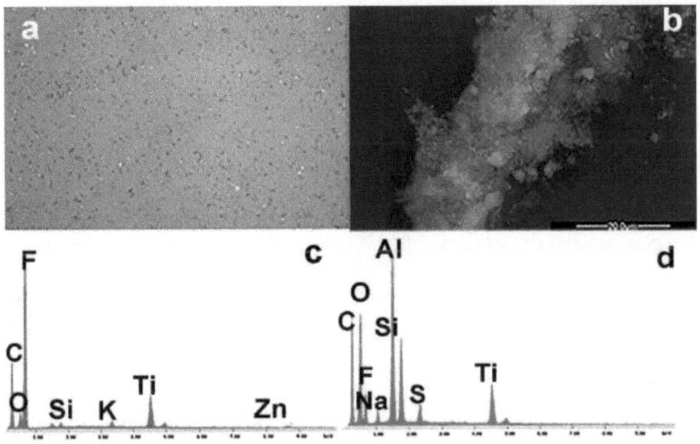

Figure 5.14 Non-stick pan. The pan's fluoride-based non-stick layer matrix containing mineral micro- (aluminium silicate) and titania (titanium dioxide) nanoparticles.

5.5 Drugs

The ideal drug should be effective on anyone and should have no side effects.

The ideal drug should only contain the active substance, at most diluted in definitely harmless media as, for example, water.

Unfortunately, the ideal drug does not exist.

Pharmakon (φάρμακον), the ancient Greek name for 'drug', means remedy but means poison as well. And there is no drug which is not, with many and huge variations, a poison.

The activity of a drug depends on a great number of variables, one of which is the extreme complexity of the animal man together with the far-from-negligible difference there is between individual and individual and also in the same individual over time. So, a drug can be more or less occasionally beneficial for one, indifferent for someone else and harmful for a third subject. Let us just take as an easy example – caffeine, a very common natural compound used also in many medicaments: there is someone who takes large amounts of it every day without showing any particular effect; others who have a headache if they abuse it; others who are kept awake the whole night if they only take a drop of coffee and, finally, people who can't sleep if they do not drink their cup before bedtime. But of substances which behave in a very different way, as is the case of caffeine, there are many. In fact, almost all of them, although in most cases the differences are not so extreme, with the due exceptions of allergic reactions.

Paradoxical effects are very well known by pharmacologists and toxicologists. A paradoxical effect or paradoxical reaction is the result of the administration of a medical drug, opposite to the effect which would normally be expected – for example, pain caused by a pain relief medication, suicidal compulsions from anti-depressants or the so-called Eagle effect [5–9].[a]

So, what is currently considered to be a good drug is one which is statistically effective (and beneficial) to a majority of subjects.

It should be added that side effects may occur any time, and it is not so rare that they become evident only after a long time: odds which are particularly critical for those who take the same drug in a chronic way. In fact, however long and accurate a trial is, it will never cover all the possibilities which a drug encounters, and, like it or not, after all, to a greater or lesser extent, anyone taking a drug is a guinea pig.

It can also be interesting to remember how not too seldom a placebo has a better effect than a drug aimed to treat a certain disease. The reason for this apparent oddity is easily explained considering the concept of homeostasis, that is, the self-regulating processes by which man, as well as any living being, tends to maintain biological stability while adjusting to conditions which are the best possible for the continuation of life in a state of well-being. At the same time, it must be remembered that all pharmaceuticals are also poisons (see their Greek etymology) and, as such, are potentially harmful as well as hopefully beneficial. It may happen that the damage outweighs the benefit, and therefore, in those cases, it is much more convenient to let the organism intervene according to the homeostasis just mentioned. In short, it may happen that letting nature work is more advantageous than replacing her.

---

[a]The effect originally referred to the reduced antibacterial effect of penicillin at high doses, a paradoxical effect because the effectiveness of an antibiotic generally rises with increasing drug concentration.

To make matters more complicated, there is the crossover effect of drugs, something which, especially when the medicaments administered to the same patient are relatively numerous, is very hard, if not utterly impossible, to predict.

Nowadays, drugs are not prepared on the spot, immediately and on request. The use of galenic preparations is also rapidly declining, and almost all of today's medicaments are industrial products which are made to be manageable for the caregiver and for those who take them; which must be movable and storable for a long-enough time, maintaining unchanged their characteristics; and which must be the least possible sensitive to environmental conditions, for example, those relating to temperature and humidity. In addition to that, the drug should not be too unpleasant for those who use it. So, a lot of substances which have nothing to do with the active ingredient but are necessary to accomplish all those results are added, and it is not impossible that those substances exert some side effect.

A practical problem concerning drugs is the presence of the same active ingredient in products with different commercial names. So, it happens that the same patient takes too high doses of the same drug, believing that it is something different. This occurs frequently when the patient turns to several specialists who do not know about each other and who prescribe the same active ingredient or the set of the same active ingredients with different brand names. Just to give an example relating to an active ingredient used and abused, having to write a book on the subject, we found that in Italy paracetamol is present 470 times.

Anyone taking drugs as tablets necessarily takes substances as micro- and nanoparticles added on purpose to dilute the active ingredient, to ensure that the drug does not break before being taken but disintegrates once it has entered the body, to make the product pleasant to the eye and so on. Also gelatin capsules and syrups may contain particulate excipients as an addition. Thus, particles such as those of talc or titanium dioxide are swallowed together with the active ingredient.

To our knowledge, a study has never been conducted showing that the amount of excipients taken is equivalent to that in any way eliminated. Therefore, it is not known whether something remains in the organism, where and how much. As a rule, the excipients in the form of particles are evaluated exclusively from a chemical point of view, and according to this criterion, their reactivity is negligible or, in practical terms, zero. But if one looks at them from the nanopathological point of view, it is clear that those particles are foreign bodies which necessarily behave as such. And the fact becomes particularly important for those who must take a drug in a chronic or, in any case, in a prolonged way over time. But now micro- and nanoparticles are also used in many sunscreens to block UVA and UVB rays. In the cosmetics industry, they are used in toothpaste, lipsticks, creams, ointments and powders, and there are many industrial foods which contain them as a deliberate addition, if not as ignored pollutants. Though the Food and Drug Administration (FDA) has approved titanium dioxide particles for food, drugs and cosmetics, there is no actual evidence about their safety.

On top of it, a number of drugs, or, at least, a substantial number among those we had a chance to check, are polluted by solid, inorganic particles whose effects depend on many variables, the most important of which are due to the class the medicament belongs to. Particles in a cream to be spread on the skin may prove to be not particularly dangerous but not so, as just mentioned, for particles polluting a medication taken orally. Much more dangerous are the particle-polluted medicaments taken by aerosol and, to the maximum of dangerousness, those administered as an injectable solution. Of course, since they are pollutants, they cannot be expected to be listed in the technical data sheet prepared by the manufacturer. In short, they are there but they are ignored.

We have no idea where those particles polluting drugs come from, be it from the raw materials used, from the technical procedures or from a production environment which is not perfectly clean. To be able to give an answer and, maybe, suggest solutions, we should be permitted to inspect the producer's facilities, something which we have never been allowed to do. What is certain is that the checks which should be carried out by the manufacturers and, a fortiori, by the relevant public bodies are, to say the least, insufficient.

The following three figures (Figs. 5.15, 5.16 and 5.17) show electron microscopy images of particulate matter contained in the drugs rafton, torvast and lansoprazole, respectively.

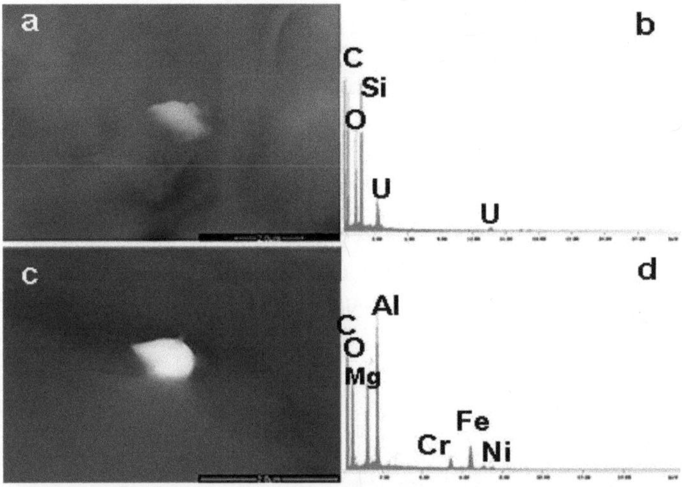

(a)

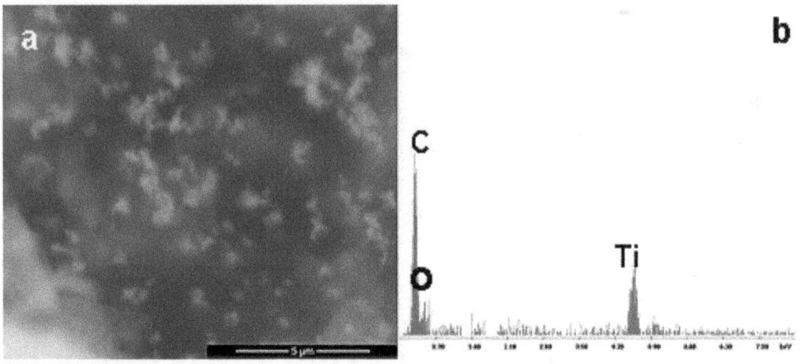

(b)

Figure 5.15 Rafton is a corticosteroid drug (budesonide) in the form of capsules used as a symptomatic against chronic diarrhea and in mild forms of Crohn's disease. Regardless of the presence of particles used as an excipient without knowing their actual fate, that of almost usual steel and non-unusual titanium, the most notable presence is the uranium component in some particles.

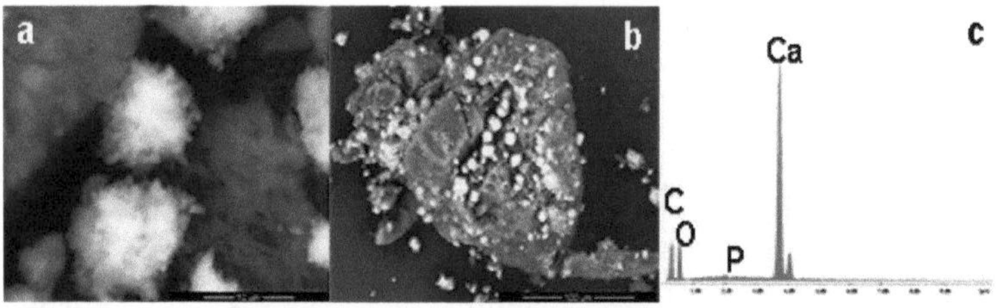

Figure 5.16 Torvast is a statin administered as tablet which is used to lower blood lipid levels. The particles found are calcium-based with dimensions ranging from the fraction of a micron to a hundred microns. Being a drug which is taken orally, it must be considered that the gastrointestinal system is permeable to large particles, and it is not known whether those we detected are biodegradable and, if so, in how long. If the particle takes a relatively long time to degrade, it may have time enough to trigger the inflammatory reaction.

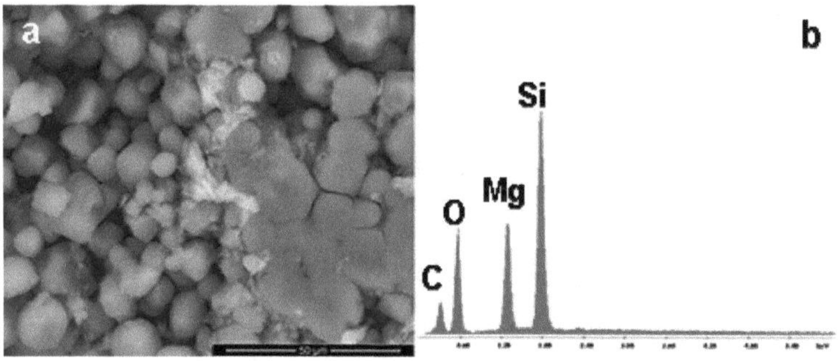

Figure 5.17 Lansoprazole, sold under the commercial name of Lansox, is a medication which reduces stomach acid. Talc (Mg-Si) is used as an excipient.

Appendix: Why Chelation Therapy Is Ineffective with Nanoparticles

A relatively high number of large molecules (e.g. proteins, polysaccharides and polynucleic acids) called ligands, due to certain chemical characteristics of theirs, can bind a metal ion in a cyclic or ring structure in a kind of pincer action. Chelating agents, particularly, though not exclusively, salts of ethylenediaminetetraacetic acid (EDTA), are widely used in medical practice to treat metal poisoning. Their administration, although currently used without too many precautions, is quite critical and not easy to dose correctly. Chemical selectivity as to the element meant to be eliminated is not particularly high, so, in addition to affecting the toxic cation to be removed, medical chelation involves elements which, in trace or in larger quantities, are beneficial to the organism, such as calcium, iron, zinc, magnesium and selenium, which, except in the case of poisoning by one of those elements, should remain undisturbed. Side effects, the quickest of which to become manifest is in general a feeling of fatigue, are therefore numerous; some of them are even very serious, and the use of chelation agents should be reserved to strict necessity and limited as much as possible in time.

It must be added that chelating agents cannot negotiate the lipophilic cellular membrane, and therefore, they cannot act against intracellular poisoning. For example, in a biological environment (e.g. the blood), organic mercury is lipophilic and can easily enter the cells, settling in the cytoplasm and then in the mitochondria as Hg^{2+}. Hydrophobic agents are sometimes added to chelators to have them enter the cell, but their efficacy is controversial.

In any case, chelators are useless against inorganic, solid, insoluble particles. In fact, they can sequester only ions, while the metallic and non-metallic elements composing particles are generally part of alloys or crystals or are amorphous structures. Furthermore, a particle is generally stable and, however, is much bigger than an atom. To make an easily understandable example, trying to hook a particle with a chelating agent is like trying to grab an elephant with eyelash tweezers. So, considering their actual efficacy and their long list of contraindications and side effects, before administering a chelation therapy it is mandatory to understand the nature of the intoxication meant to be treated. Then, once the chelation therapy has started, it is essential to check the patient about the chemical balance of the trace elements present in his/her body to avoid the risk of stealing something indispensable.

Regardless of actual chelation, several different remedies which have nothing to do with that chemical process are proposed to free the body from inorganic pollutants, even particulate ones. Zeolite, a family of microporous, alumino-silicate minerals, is one of them (Fig. 5.18). Of the more than 200 different formulas existing, about 40 are of natural geological origin and they are capable of accommodating in their structure a wide variety of cations. On their 'purifying' properties, at least for some of them, there is a certain episodic literature, but in fact, there is no evidence relating to their effectiveness, especially as for micro- and nanoparticles. And nothing can be found in the literature to demonstrate that all the product ingested is actually eliminated and how.

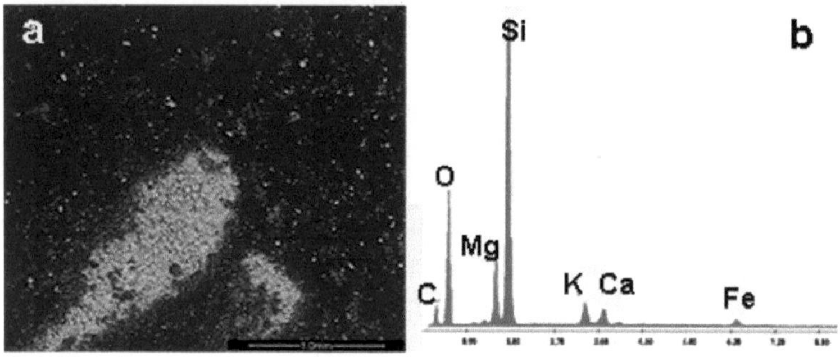

Figure 5.18 Zeolites are microporous, alumino-silicate minerals of volcanic origin with a structure which somehow recalls that of activated carbon. The large surface in relation to their volume suggests an ability to trap substances harmful to the body. There is a relatively large amount of episodic literature which reports success in cases of the most diverse pathologies. To our knowledge, however, not enough extensive studies exist over time to check whether the benefits have been preserved and whether side effects have occurred if not all the zeolite introduced into the body was then eliminated in the stool or in any other way. In that case, zeolite would be a solid, inorganic and non-biodegradable foreign body.

In our experience, getting rid of micro- and nanoparticles when they have been captured by tissues is something which no drugs have shown to be able to do.

References

1. Gatti, A., Tossini, D., Gambarelli, A., Montanari, S., and Capitani F. (2009). Environmental scanning electron microscope and energy dispersive system investigation of inorganic micro- and nano-particles in bread and biscuits. *Crit. Rev. Food Sci. Nutr.*, **49**(3), pp. 275–282.
2. Merliss, R. R. (1971). Talc-treated rice and Japanese stomach cancer. *Science*, **173**(4002), pp. 1141–1142.
3. Park, E. J., Bae, E., Yi, J., Kim, Y., Choi, K., Lee, S. H., Yoon, J., Lee, B. C., and Park, K. (2010). Repeated-dose toxicity and inflammatory responses

in mice by oral administration of silver nanoparticles. *Environ. Toxicol. Pharmacol.*, **30**(2), pp. 162–168.

4. Musselman, H. A. D. (1948). The rate of bactericidal action of penicillin in vitro as a function of its concentration, and its paradoxically reduced activity at high concentrations against certain organisms. *J. Exp. Med.*, **88**(1), pp. 99–131.
5. Yourassowsky, E., Vander Linden, M. P., Lismont, M. J., and Schoutens, E. (1978). Qualitative study of paradoxical zone phenomenon of penicillins against 17 bacterial species of clinical importance. *Chemotherapy*, **24**(2), pp. 92–96.
6. Stevens, D. L., Gibbons, A. E., Bergstrom, R., and Winn, V. (1988). The Eagle effect revisited: efficacy of clindamycin, erythromycin, and penicillin in the treatment of streptococcal myositis. *J. Infect. Dis.*, **158**(1), pp. 23–28.
7. Pollard, A. J., McCracken, G. H., and Finn, A. (2004). *Hot Topics in Infection and Immunity in Children*. Springer, UK, p. 187.
8. Ikeda, Y., Fukuoka, Y.m Motomura, K., Yasuda, T., and Nishino, T. (1990). Paradoxical activity of beta-lactam antibiotics against Proteus vulgaris in experimental infection in mice. *Antimicrob. Agents Chemother.*, **34**(1), pp. 94–97.
9. Hugo, W. B. and Russel, A. D. (2004). *Pharmaceutical Microbiology*, 7th ed. Denyer, S. P., Hodges, N. A., and Gorman, S. P., eds. Blackwell Science, USA, p. 188.

Chapter 6

The Injection Pathway and Other Entry Channels

If inhalation and ingestion are by far the most common entry channels into the organism, they are not the only ones.

As will be explained later in this book, injectable drugs may contain particles as pollutants, or, for example, in the case of colloidal gold, nanoparticles are administered purposefully as a remedy against arthritis. It must be clear that, as they are administered by injection, none of those foreign bodies can be eliminated.

As to entry channels which are not ingestion and inhalation/respiration and as to medicines, once we had the case of a subject who had stainless-steel particles in his lungs coming from polluted nasal drops he had used for years.

What may look an unusual entry was the one we came across a few years ago: an entry due to adsorption through an epithelial tissue (Fig. 6.1).

An alcohol-based mouthwash containing zinc salts had been used for decades by a patient. Alcohol had made the mouth mucosa particularly permeable, so that the partially hydrolysed zinc salt could penetrate the tissue. In the long run, the presence of salt had become supersaturated and zinc had precipitated in the form of particles inside the tongue, where we found it. That case may be seen as borderline, since the particles had not entered directly as such but had formed inside the tissue using the element made available by the salt contained in the drug. Of course, those particles could have

Advances in Nanopathology: From Vaccines to Food
Antonietta Morena Gatti and Stefano Montanari

ISBN 978-981-4877-29-9 (Hardcover), 978-1-003-05622-5 (eBook)
www.jennystanford.com

been present also in all oral cavity's tissues, but the only sample we had available was the tongue muscle (Fig. 6.1).

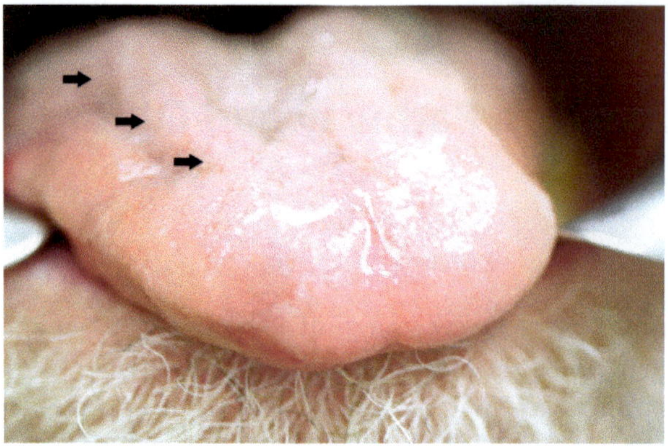

(a)

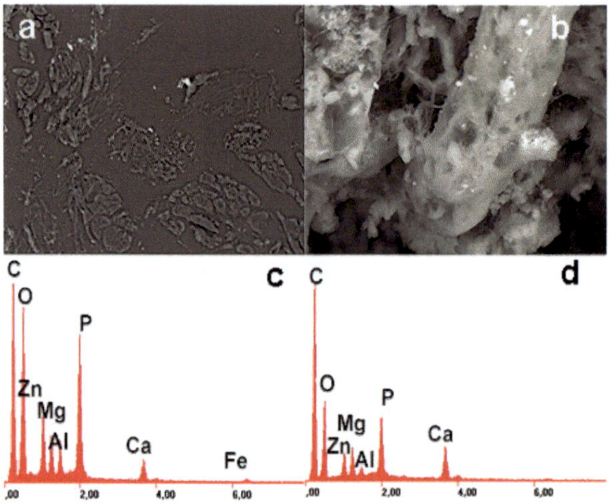

(b)

Figure 6.1 Asymmetrical tongue. The images represent the (a) asymmetrical (black arrows) surface of the tongue and (b) the biopsy of the right side of the tongue and the zinc precipitates identified inside.

The patient had a diagnosis of amyotrophic lateral syndrome.

Many cosmetics, for example, sunscreens, are plus micro- and nanoparticles, and though we don't have experience enough in that field, having not had the chance to analyse a sufficient number of specimens and human cases, we think that the possibility of their introduction in the body and to what extent cannot be ruled out before all the appropriate research is completed.

6.1 Biocompatibility of What Is Introduced in the Body by Injection

It is only obvious that the compounds injected in the body must be compatible with the blood components. That means that they must not interact either chemically or physically with its components and must not have actions which go beyond what they are specifically required to do.

6.2 Vaccines

This book is not meant to cover the use and efficacy of vaccines nor the many disputes in this regard which are often heated and not always properly founded. Much has been written claiming completely opposing arguments. Much has been influenced by the enormous economic interests which investments in vaccines entail. Much has been censored.

Vaccination or something similar to it is a very old medical practice: the Chinese and the Indians employed *variolation* (administration of infected material taken from human patients suffering from smallpox) centuries before Edward Jenner did with the bovine variety of the pathogen, and the practice was also in use in Africa, in Persia and in Turkey long before being spread in Europe and, much later, in America. The aim of that pharmacological treatment based on the observation of immunity acquired by those who had fallen ill and had recovered was that of inducing immunity to a certain disease. For many centuries it was only smallpox, through the administration of the pathogen in a hopefully harmless form. As a matter of fact, the practice was not always risk-free and mortality was far from negligible, but it is more than probable that the practice was, after all, advantageous.

Whatever the philosophical and cultural approach to vaccination, it must be recalled that vaccines are drugs. So, like all drugs, they are not equally active on all individuals, whatever is meant by activity, and they have contraindications (e.g. immunodepression, an ongoing pathological state, already acquired immunity, allergy to one or more components) and side effects. And, in particular, the duration of the immunity which may be acquired through vaccines is limited to some years, and thus, unlike what happens with the naturally acquired disease, booster doses are generally required. For that reason, not to make promises which can't be kept charging vaccines of expectations which go beyond their means, the concept of the so-called 'herd immunity'[a] should be revised in a more objective and rational way and more closely to facts.

Like all drugs in use today, vaccines also must be acceptably stable, acceptably resistant to temperature variations and have a long-enough shelf life. So, as happens with most drugs, substances are added which have nothing to do with the active ingredient. Moreover, vaccines contain processing residues such as proteins, red blood cells and mercury, a metal which is added more and more rarely in the final formulation but which remains in trace from production processes. As an example, Sanofi Pasteur declared that their quadrivalent influenza vaccine Fluzone meant to be administered to subjects from 6 months or older contains 12.5 mcg of mercury/0.25 dose for ages 6–35 months and 25 mcg of mercury/0.5 ml dose for ages older than 36 months.

For many reasons, not a few of which completely foreign to medicine, it is hardly possible to find today a more controversial topic in medicine than vaccines.

As already mentioned, it is not our intention to discuss here the many problems involving that type of product: how the pathologies are chosen, the differences in choice between country and country, often neighbouring countries where there are completely different obligations or where the obligation does not exist at all, how vaccines are produced, how they are tested (just a hint will be given in a few pages), what their real efficacy is and what their side effects, how they are controlled, how they are administered, how people who undergo vaccination are informed, how they are medically checked before vaccination, how side effects are collected and catalogued,

[a]Herd immunity is a form of indirect protection from an infectious pathology which is argued to occur when a large percentage of a population has become immune to an infection, thus disrupting, hindering or slowing the spread of disease.

etc. It should only be remembered that vaccines are drugs and that drugs, taking for granted their harmlessness as an act of faith, are administered only when necessary if one wants to act according to good medical practice.

Our only aim here is to report what we found in those products, analysing them as we usually do.

We started to check vaccines on the request of the German University of Mainz. The problem reported was a painful swelling at the injection site which often occurred in those who underwent vaccination, and thus, the university sent us, together with the vaccine samples, and also the skin biopsies.

Much to our surprise, we found both kinds of samples polluted by solid, inorganic particles. We repeated the analyses several times, since we could not believe that an injectable drug, least of all a vaccine, could be polluted, but all tests gave the same results.

Sometime later, we were asked to analyse a vaccine administered to a young soldier who had died of cancer. The postmortem sample of the cancerous tissue we checked showed the presence of micro- and nanoparticles typical of many similar cases, and also the vaccine proved to be polluted by solid, inorganic particles, but in that case, the pollutants we found were entirely different. If the presence of particles in a cancer could be considered to be 'normal', as we detected in a great number of cases, it was not so in a vaccine. However, as regards that particular case, there was no evidence that the particles contained in the vaccine were responsible for the soldier's illness and death.

Later, the Italian University of Parma sent us a student who was preparing her doctoral thesis and with her we analysed 19 types of vaccines. All of them proved to be polluted by different solid, inorganic particles.

Now, at the time of writing these pages, the types of different vaccines we have tested are 45. For some of them it was only one samples; for others it was several, in some circumstances obtained from different sources and produced in different years. None of them proved to be free from particulate pollution with the sole exception of the only veterinary vaccine we analysed: Feligen (Virbac S.r.l.), a vaccine meant for the immunisation of cats against feline rhinotracheitis virus, feline calcivirus and feline panleucopaenia virus.

It is only obvious that no drug should contain pollutants, whatever they are. A fortiori, there should be no fragments of matter evidently incompatible with the human body in an injectable product. The problem is further aggravated by the fact that many vaccines are injected into newborn babies and are administered repeatedly over time.

We have already pointed out that one of the basic principles of toxicology is that poisons exert a mutually synergistic action and the higher the number of poisons which act simultaneously, the more difficult it grows, until it becomes impossible, to guess what their final effect will be.

The obvious question as far as we are directly concerned is where those particles come from. Among our many perplexities, there are the accuracy and reliability of the controls which must be carried out both by the producers and by the health authorities, and the reason why that very visible pollution is undetected or kept hidden or, when this is reported and reaches some publicity, an attempt is made to minimise its importance and danger, when not to deny its existence. One thing is certain: regardless of any consideration and attempt at justification, those particles may not be there.

Leaving aside the pollution from particulate matter for a moment, it is enough to read the technical data sheets of any vaccines to see how those drugs contain substances which are poorly or not at all compatible with the physiology of the human body. Among these substances there are, for example, formaldehyde, aluminium with some of its compounds and various antibiotics to which different subjects are allergic. But, more than once, there are also fragments of human DNA from aborted foetal tissues (in no less than 30 types of different vaccines), red blood cells, viruses (e.g. SV40 in the anti-poliomyelitis vaccine), pesticides (e.g. glyphosate), pork jelly, etc.

Among the many possible examples of non-harmless substances contained in vaccines and listed as components by the producers themselves, formaldehyde, whose carcinogenicity is well known, can be listed [1–9].

To this can be added aluminium, the most common adjuvant used in large quantities in vaccines. Its toxicity, especially at the neurological level, is perfectly known for several years, so much so that for some time its use in the kitchen and in cosmetics has been strongly discouraged. Curiously enough, however, aluminium is hardly mentioned when is administered along with vaccines [9–65]. It is also necessary to consider how aluminium is injected even into premature babies.

But, apart from pollutants and what has just been mentioned, vaccines also contain substances which can cause even violent allergic reactions. Among these there are substances which come from the eggs of birds and antibiotics such as neomycin and kanamycin, however not recommended in children.

It should be added that the candidates for vaccination are never checked in advance for their ability to tolerate these substances. Nor is it practically possible to do so in infants, particularly if premature.

Thus, if we look at the issue from a coldly scientific point of view, it is impossible not to wonder about the harmlessness of those drugs and the blind way they are administered, not only without the most basic preliminary controls, but even to people who have already suffered from infectious diseases like, for instance, measles, becoming naturally immune.

It is often said that vaccines are meticulously and thoroughly tested.

As is the case with any drug, to be such and to give acceptable answers the test must be carried out in a double-blind fashion. If the drug is intended to combat a specific disease, the highest possible number of homogeneous patients affected by that disease is taken and divided into two groups, to one of which the product under examination is administered and to the other a placebo. At the end of the test, the experimenters check and count how many subjects of each group have recovered from the disease and, thus, the effectiveness of the medicament is determined. This is virtually impossible with vaccines. In the first place, the subjects on whom the experimenters have to work must necessarily be healthy and, the diseases being infectious, it is not possible to know in advance if they will fall ill, how many of them will and, in the event that sooner or later they will, in how long. Thus, to obtain a statistically acceptable result on a vaccine, and the reliability of statistics is largely linked to the amount of reliable data available and to the fact that the morbidity of infectious diseases is extremely variable and unpredictable, it is essential to work on a huge number of subjects for many years. This would require huge economic investments with a possible, but far from certain, in any case much delayed, economic return compared to what the entrepreneur desires. Since pharmaceutical companies are companies like all others and their goal is, of course, profit, none of these things is done and serious experimentation simply does not exist.

Unfortunately, this very serious deficiency is neglected both by law and by the medical class, and the information which passes to the general public is that vaccines are carefully tested.

As for safety, suffice what in 2010 the US Supreme Court ruled: 'Vaccines are unavoidably unsafe products' [66].

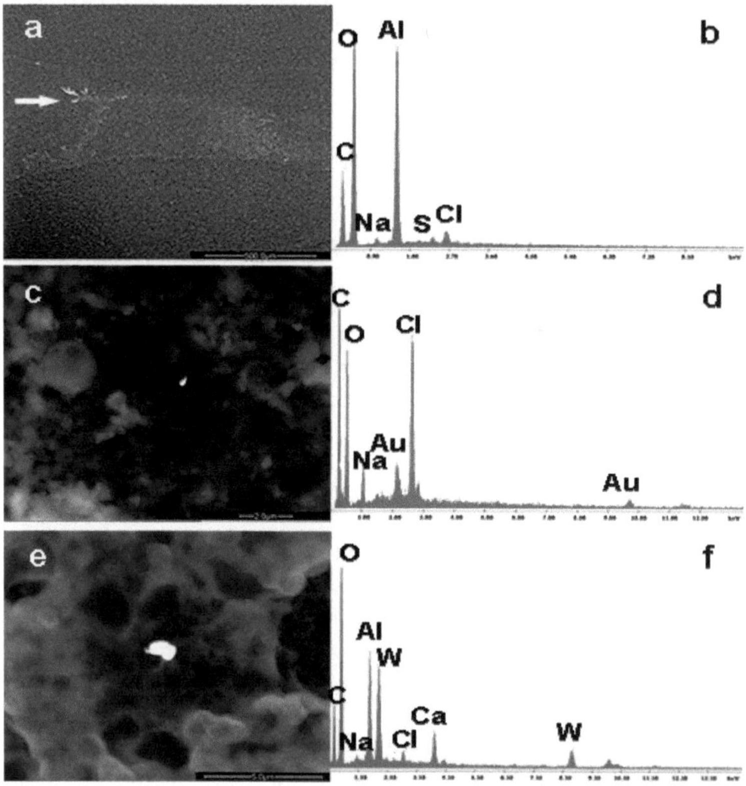

Figure 6.2 Contamination of DiTeBooster vaccine (AjVaccines, Denmark). DiTeBooster is used to vaccinate children who should not be younger than 5 and adults who have already received primary vaccination against diphtheria and tetanus. As in all the vaccines for human use which we have analysed, this too is polluted by the presence of particles of a predominantly metallic nature and quite often smaller than 1 μm in size.

It is only obvious that evaluating the toxicity of a vaccine observing for some time, often only days, the behaviour of a test animal cannot give reliable indications. A fortiori, information on efficacy cannot be expected, and this is not only because of the too small number of animals and the too short observation time but also, above all, because animals do not fall ill with diseases which are typically human, such as measles, chicken pox, rubella, etc.

Ultimately, what vaccine producers make and say is accepted as a certainty and an article of faith, and the actual guinea pigs are those who should benefit from the product.

It is sad to say that anyone who points out the obvious facts briefly described is considered an 'enemy of science', when it should be exactly the opposite. In any case, no problem can be addressed if its existence is denied a priori, however opposing a point of view, or its discussion prevented by denying or hiding facts or, even worse, by using violence.

Whatever the claims, scientific dignity must necessarily undergo a sort of never-ending trial, and a refusal or avoidance, however one tries to justify it, disqualifies the statement itself or, at the very least, cannot but raise legitimate doubts in its regard.

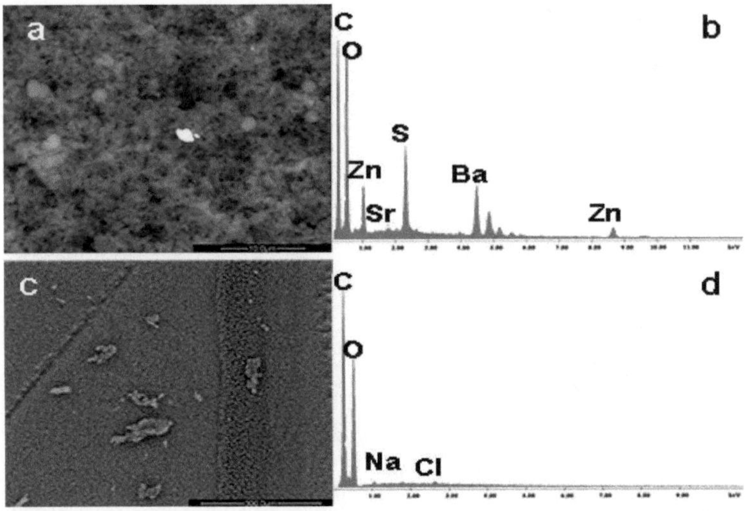

Figure 6.3 Fluad vaccine (Seqirus, Italy). It is one of many flu shots. It too has been shown to contain solid, inorganic and incompatible particles with the organism. It contains particles of barium sulphate and crystals of the saline solution.

The following images (Figs. 6.2–6.13) regard inorganic debris we have found in a 40 μl drop of some vaccines. The article 'New Quality-Control Investigations on Vaccines: Micro- and Nanocontamination (2017)' [67] has already showed the presence of particles which do not belong to the pharmaceutical formula of those vaccines nor, to be sure, of any injectable medicament. Some examples of this contamination with its chemical composition are shown but are not discussed, since we do not have any explanation to those undue presences.

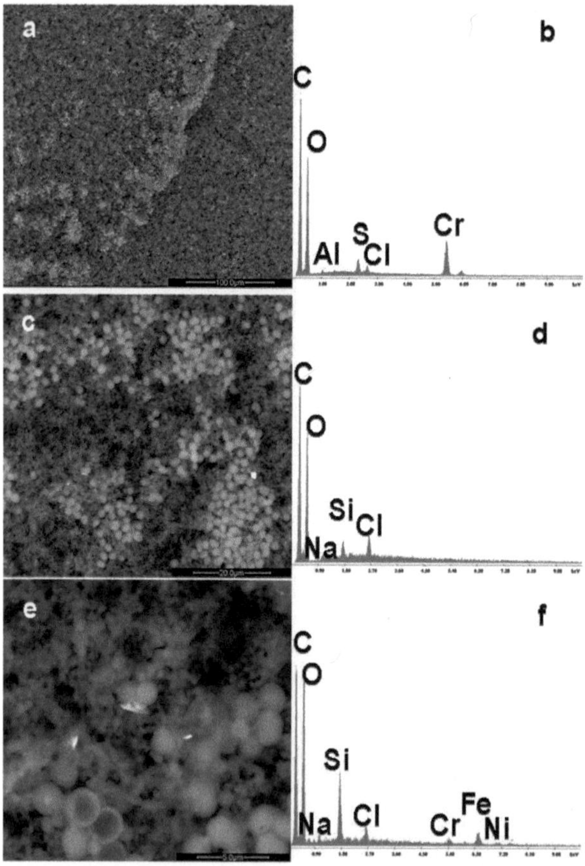

Figure 6.4 Contamination of Fluarix vaccine (GlaxoSmithKline, Great Britain). It is another of the many flu shots. It too has been shown to contain solid, inorganic and incompatible particles with the body. In this case, the particles found appear to be aluminium and stainless-steel particles and those of common household dust.

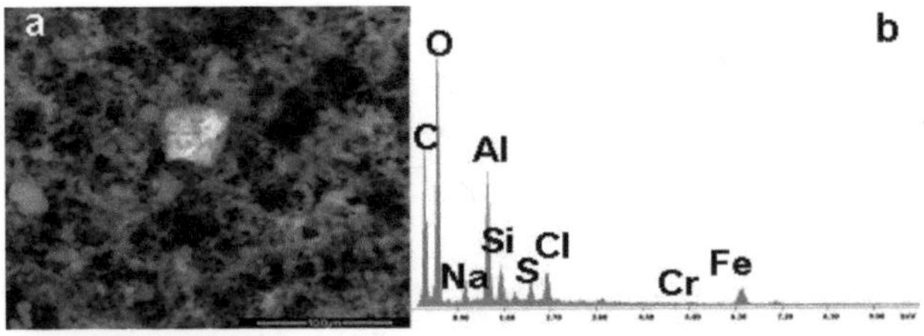

(a)

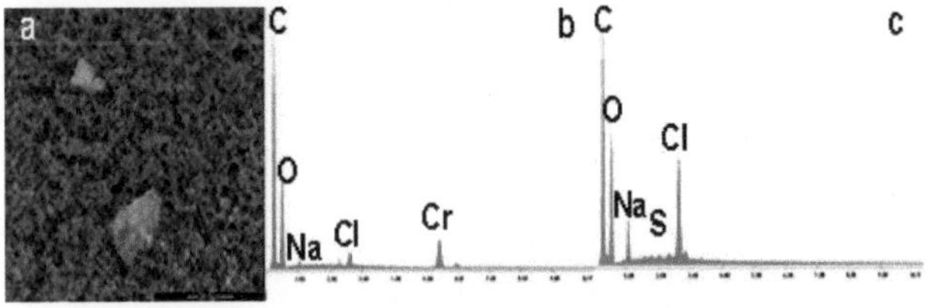

(b)

Figure 6.5 Contamination of Intanza vaccine (Sanofi Pasteur, France). It is another of the many flu shots. Considered responsible for the death of several patients, it was withdrawn from the market. Also this drug contains polluting particles, in this case also rather coarse, impossible to not detect if the product was actually controlled. It contains (a) aluminium (adjuvant) and stainless steel and (b) chromium particles. As in other cases, the sodium chloride–based particles are due to the crystallisation of that salt contained in the saline solution.

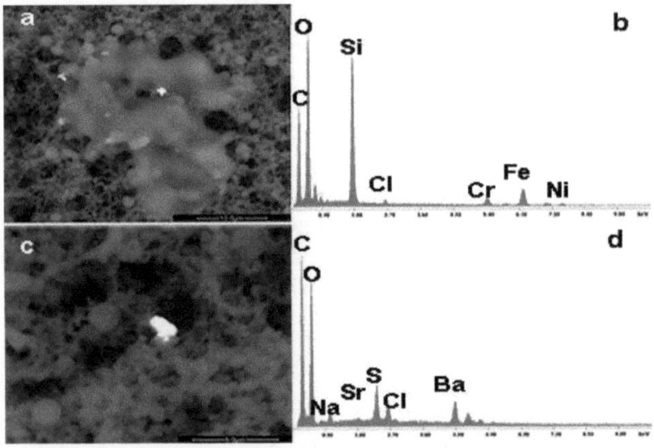

Figure 6.6 Measles vaccine (PaxVaxBerna, Switzerland). It is a measles vaccine purchased in Switzerland. Note, in addition to the barium sulphate–based particles, the majority component of silicon in those containing stainless steel (iron, chromium and nickel). It is interesting to observe the formation of proteins around these latter particles.

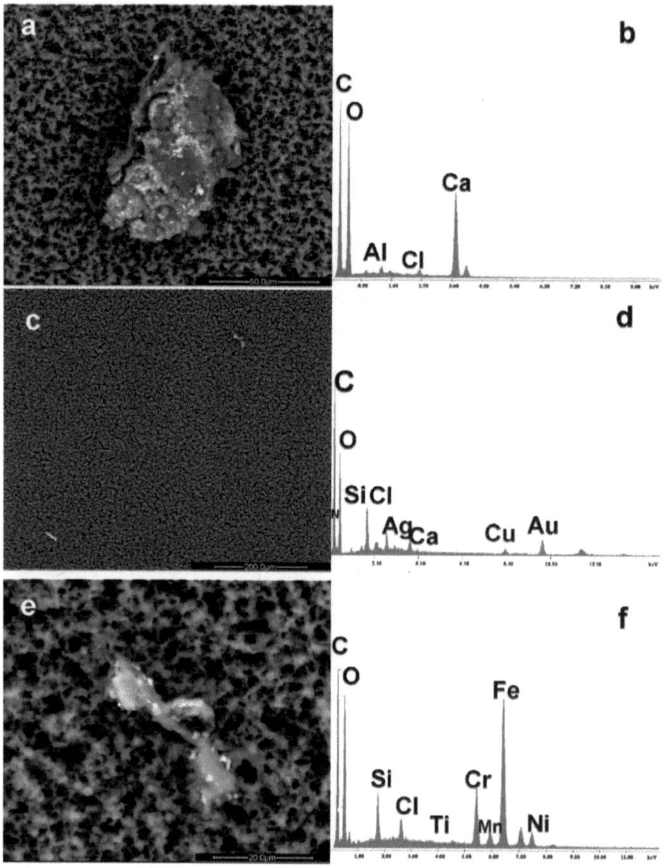

Figure 6.7 Priorix vaccine (GlaxoSmithKline, Great Britain). Priorix trivalent vaccine against measles, mumps and rubella should be used with extreme caution and, in any case, always having taken all the dictated both by good medical practice and by what the manufacturer writes. This is due to the side effects, of which, at least in our experience, a not negligible fraction of the vaccinated population suffers. The particles found in the samples we checked have a rather varied composition and include, in addition to iron, chromium and nickel (f), almost usual, also gold and silver (d) and calcium (b).

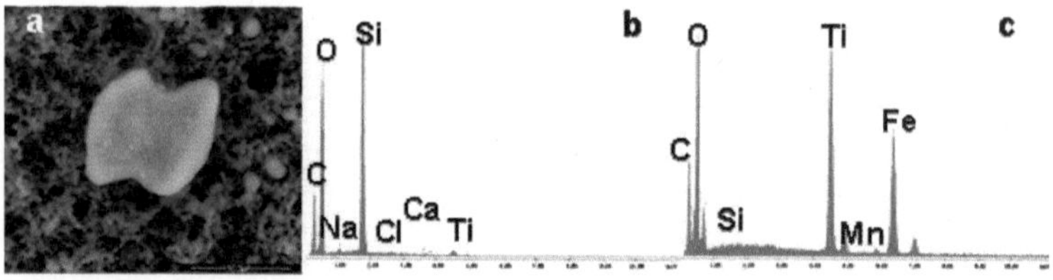

(a)

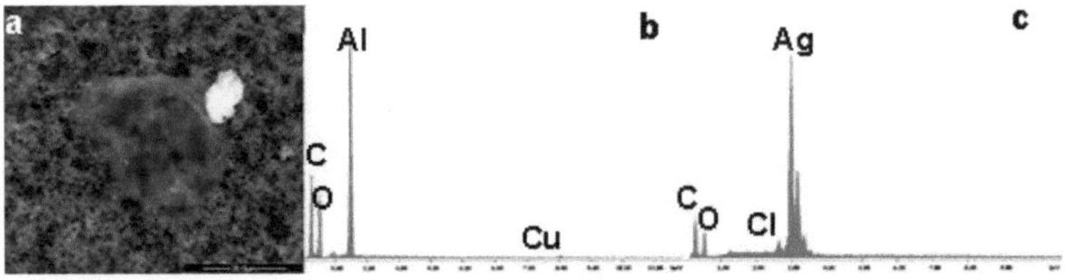

(b)

Figure 6.8 Stamaril (Sanofi Pasteur, France). It is a specific viral vaccine against yellow fever. The samples we analysed showed particle pollutants which, in some instances, were quite coarse and, therefore, impossible not to identify if a control was actually performed. (a) Silicon and titanium and (b) aluminium and silver were the major components of the particles found in the samples we analysed.

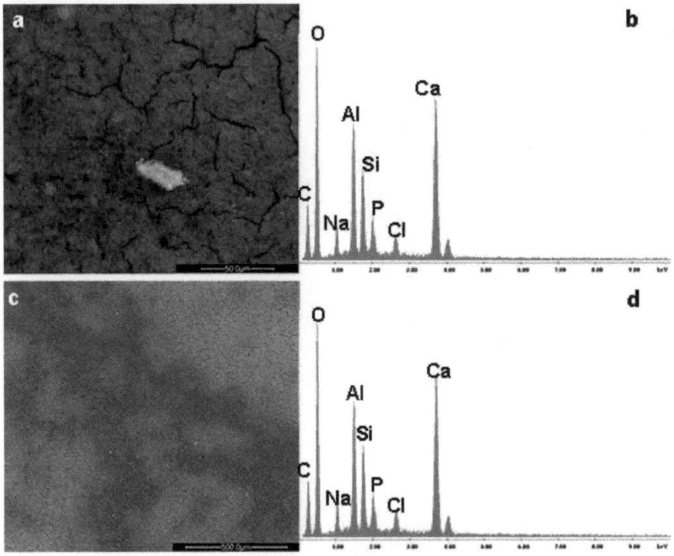

Figure 6.9 Synflorix (GlaxoSmithKline, Poland). It is a vaccine for active immunisation against invasive disease, pneumonia and acute otitis media caused by *Streptococcus pneumoniae* in infants and children from 6 weeks to 5 years of age. The manufacturer does not guarantee its safety in children who have exceeded 5 years of age. The product is conjugated to protein D (derived from non-typable *Haemophilus influenzae*), to the tetanus toxoid and to the diphtheria toxoid. Also in this case the analyses showed the presence of numerous solid polluting particles. Note, among others, that of particularly large dimensions based on calcium, aluminium and silicon. The presence of aluminium and phosphorus can be explained by what the manufacturer claims, namely that the product is adsorbed on aluminium phosphate (0.5 mg of aluminium per dose).

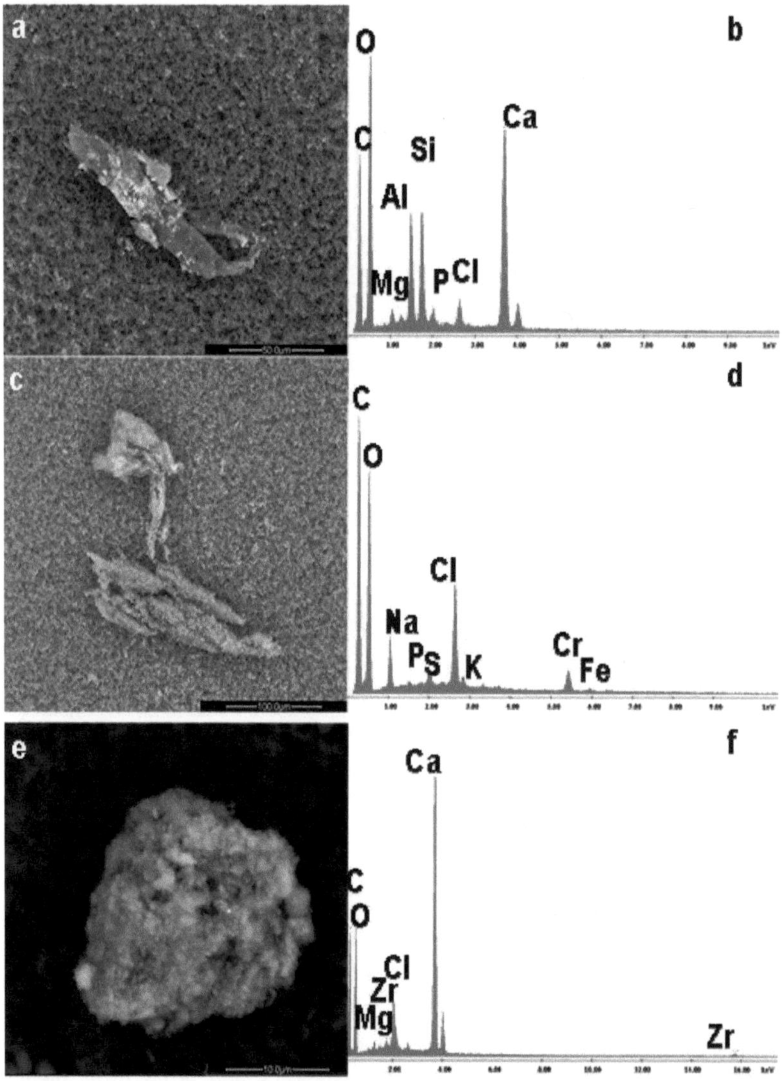

Figure 6.10 Influvac Tetra Mylan Health PTY Limited (Australia). Among the many flu vaccine samples which we have analysed, this one, purchased in Sydney (Australia), is the one which has shown the presence of coarser inorganic solid particulate, totally impossible not to detect. It is difficult to believe that the product has been actually checked. In many cases, we detected very-small-particle agglomerations. It is impossible for us to determine whether, once injected into the body, those agglomerates will remain so or will crumble into their small components.

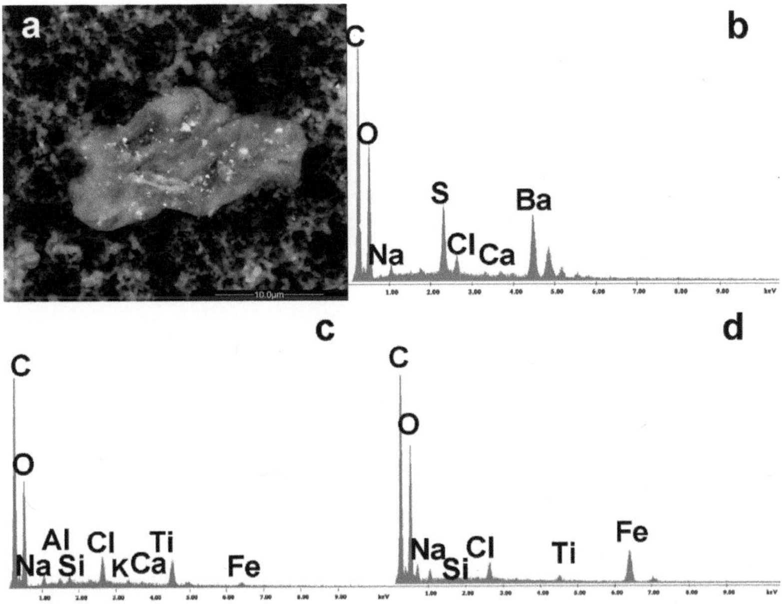

(a)

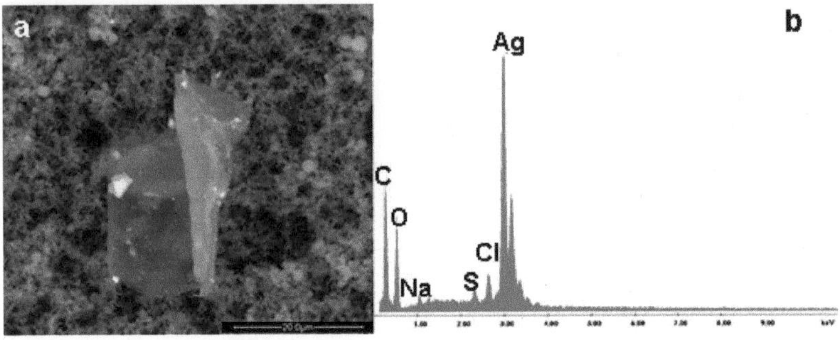

(b)

Figure 6.11 Typhim Vi vaccine (Sanofi Pasteur, Denmark). Typhim Vi is aimed at the active immunisation against typhoid fever caused by *Salmonella enterica serovar Typhi* in adults or children aged 2 years or older. Note the presence of coarse particles based on silver and others based on titanium. Also in this as in other vaccines, there is a strong component of barium and sulphur in the polluting particles.

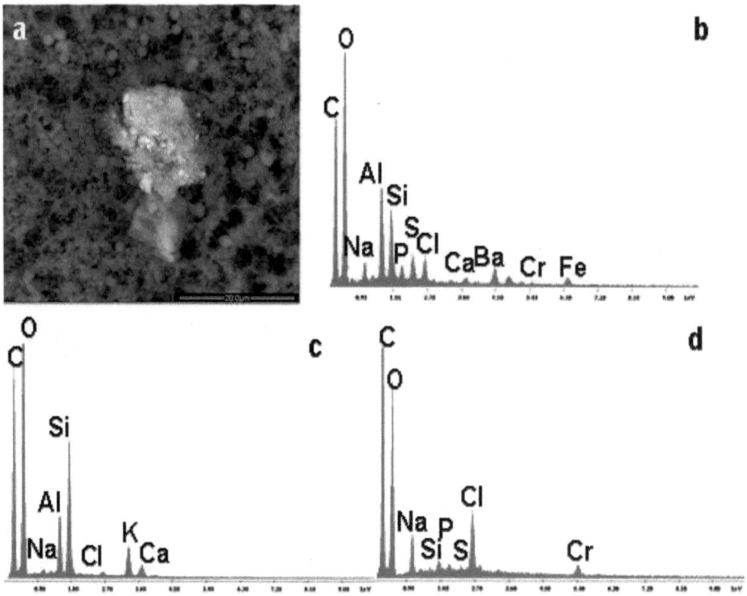

Figure 6.12 Vaxygrip vaccine (Sanofi Pasteur, Denmark). Yet another flu shot. As in all other cases, this too presents pollution from inorganic solid particles. With permission from Macro Gruppo Editoriale SRL.

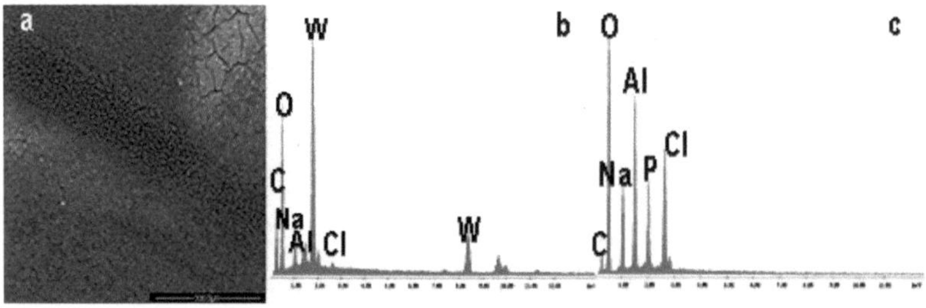

Figure 6.13 Twinrix vaccine (GlaxoSmithKline, Denmark). This is an anti-hepatitis A+B vaccine which contains as adjuvant aluminium phosphate, saline solution (sodium chloride) but also some debris of tungsten or tungsten carbide.

The presence in many vaccines of debris composed of tungsten or tungsten carbide excited our curiosity since it is a hard metal which, at our knowledge, is not used during the preparation of a drug like a vaccine. We had experience of some findings of a similar metal in cases where hard materials needed to be cold worked.

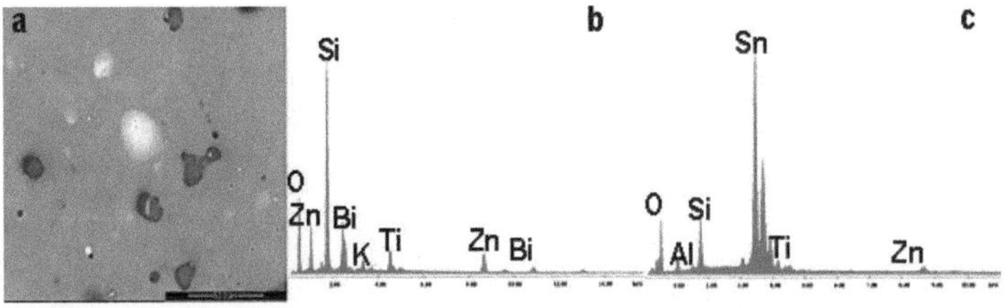

(a)

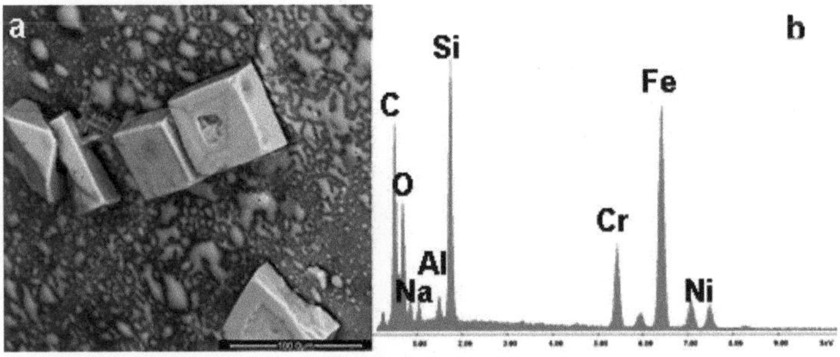

(b)

Figure 6.14 Glass of a syringe containing Typherix (GSK Australia). The images show the analyses performed on the internal glassy surface of a syringe which contained Typherix, a vaccine meant to prevent typhoid fever. The analyses showed the presence of different types of microparticles of steel, tin, zinc, titanium, bismuth, etc., debris which are inevitably injected with the vaccine (a). Silicon belongs to the composition of glass; instead iron, chromium and nickel (b) are stainless steel debris.

When we analyse a vaccine, we extract it from the syringe in which it is usually contained by passing it through the needle, thereby doing exactly what is done when the product is injected. So, if the syringe or needle is polluted by particles, it is quite possible that what we analyse and what, ultimately, enters the body of the person being vaccinated is not all contained as a pollutant in the vaccine itself but in its container and means of administration. The production of the needle starts from a long steel tube which is cut, normally on three different planes, with a tool usually made of tungsten. It is more than likely that part of the steel and tungsten particles produced by the cut enter the lumen of the needle which, as a rule, is never cleaned. As a matter of fact, tungsten and stainless steel (iron, chromium and nickel) are among the components most commonly found in our analyses performed on vaccines. As far as the glass syringe is concerned, it is hot-formed by metal tools (tungsten or tungsten carbide wire at 600°C) which can release polluting solid residues. The electron microscope images show this pollution (Figs. 6.14 and 6.15).

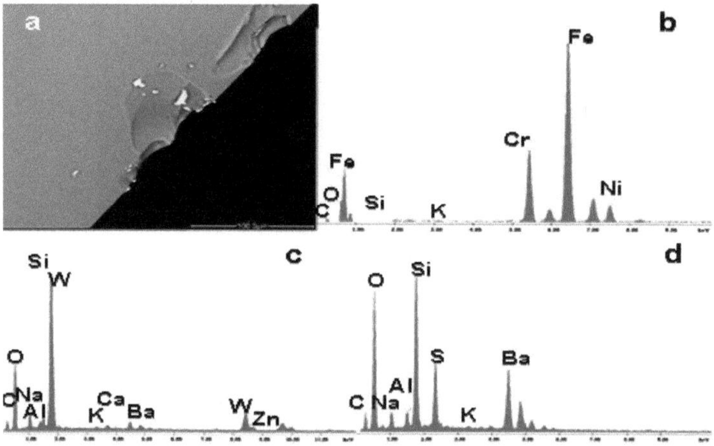

Figure 6.15 Glass of a syringe containing Priorix (GSK, Great Britain). The image shows the analyses performed on the internal glassy surface of a syringe which contained Priorix, the already mentioned vaccine meant to prevent measles, mumps and rubella. The particles detected were composed mainly of steel, tungsten, sulphur and barium.

When particulate matter is injected, it can stay at the puncture site, causing a local, inflammatory reaction, or it can be carried by the blood or lymph circulation virtually anywhere throughout the body. One of the possibilities is the passage from mother to foetus, and also for that reason vaccinating a pregnant woman may prove particularly risky.

6.3 Sudden Infant Death Syndrome

SIDS is an acronym for sudden infant death syndrome, a condition referring to the unexpected death of children under the age of one year, often between the second and fourth months of life, which occurs during sleep. The syndrome has been known for decades and has never found a definite explanation. The autopsies which the corpses of the children have undergone have never revealed anything which could be called abnormal, except for some rare cases such as that of a 7-month-old girl in whose brain, in the *area postrema*, the area at the base of the fourth ventricle, characterised by a great vascularity and outside the blood–brain barrier, evident traces of a household insecticide were found [68].

Finding nothing in the short clinical history of the baby or any specific cause, the most disparate reasons came up, from the prone position of the child in the cradle (but there are no reliable data reporting how many of the dead children were sleeping in that position) to alleged maturation defects of the brain circuits which govern the awakening of children, especially in dangerous conditions such as oxygen deficiency during respiratory infections (but also in this case, not a few babies who died in the cradle suffered from those infections or, however, of other pathologies).

Mortality rates vary significantly by population.

At the time of writing these notes (early 2020), thanks to the collaboration with the Italian foundation Lino Rossi which gives us the samples, we are analysing according to our electron microscopy technique some brain samples from children who died of SIDS.

All our analyses on autopsic brains showed the presence of mainly metallic foreign bodies which, being electrically conductive, may have interfered with the electrical activity of the nervous tissue.

A particularly interesting finding was that of 'petrified' cells where silicon was present, somehow recalling the chemical phenomenon which occurs in the petrifaction of trees. We do not yet have the opportunity to put forward any hypothesis in this regards, and we merely report the results of our observations.

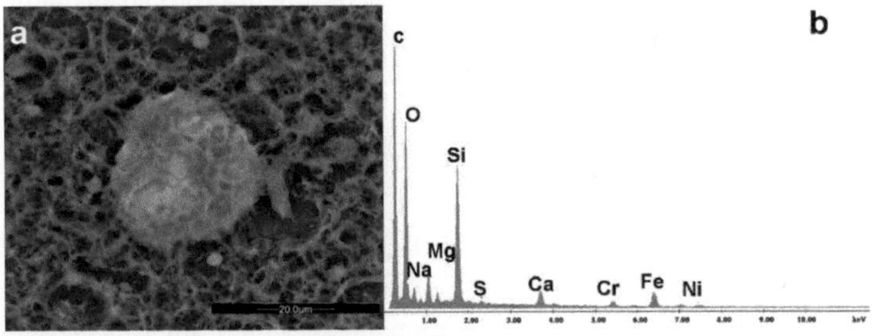

Figure 6.16 Baby's brain. The image shows part of a baby's brain with a cell which is completely transformed in its silicon content.

6.4 Sexually Transmissible Diseases by Particles

That sexually transmitted diseases exist has been known for centuries. Viruses and bacteria are the accused and often the actual culprits.

Our research has shown that another pathogen exists, and this is constituted by inorganic micro- and nanoparticles which are found more and more often in the seminal fluid of those who are in contact with pollution, and this regardless of its source.

As will be illustrated in the next chapter, these particles modify the proteins of the seminal fluid, causing reactions at the level of the mucous membranes. Furthermore, precisely because of the inflammation of the mainly vaginal and anal mucous membranes, their permeability increases, leaving an easier passage for particles.

This must be taken into account when evaluating the biocompatibility of a substance made of nanoparticles, as is the case with nanotechnological products, especially those used in medicine. Among the most used products, vaginal plugs and internal vaginal pads have never been evaluated from this point of view. Biocompatibility, in fact, is different and can vary much according to the tissue with which those particles come into contact.

References

1. U.S. Environmental Protection Agency, Office of Air and Radiation (1989). *Report to Congress on Indoor Air Quality*, Volume II: Assessment and Control of Indoor Air Pollution.
2. International Agency for Research on Cancer (2006). *IARC Monographs on the Evaluation of Carcinogenic Risks to Humans* (88) Formaldehyde, 2-Butoxyethanol and 1-tert-Butoxypropan-2-ol. Retrieved June 10, 2011, from: http://monographs.iarc.fr/ENG/Monographs/vol88/index.phpExit Disclaimer.
3. National Toxicology Program (2011). *Report on Carcinogens*, 12th ed. Department of Health and Human Services, Public Health Service, National Toxicology Program. http://ntp.niehs.nih.gov/go/roc12.
4. Hauptmann, M., Stewart, P. A., and Lubin, J. H., et al. (2009). Mortality from lymphohematopoietic malignancies and brain cancer among embalmers exposed to formaldehyde. *J. Natl. Cancer Inst.*, **101**(24), pp. 1696–1708, [PubMed Abstract].

5. Hauptmann, M., Lubin, J. H., Stewart, P. A., Hayes, R. B., and Blair, A. (2003). Mortality from lymphohematopoietic malignancies among workers in formaldehyde industries. *J. Natl. Cancer Inst.*, **95**(21), pp. 1615–1623, [PubMed Abstract].
6. Beane Freeman, L., Blair, A., Lubin, J. H., et al. (2009). Mortality from lymphohematopoietic malignancies among workers in formaldehyde industries: The National Cancer Institute Cohort. *J. Natl. Cancer Inst.*, **101**(10), pp. 751–761, [PubMed Abstract].
7. Pinkerton, L. E., Hein, M. J., and Stayner, L. T. (2004). Mortality among a cohort of garment workers exposed to formaldehyde: an update. *Occup. Environ. Med.*, **61**, pp. 193–200, [PubMed Abstract].
8. Coggon, D., Harris, E. C., Poole, J., and Palmer, K. T. (2003). Extended follow-up of a cohort of British chemical workers exposed to formaldehyde. *J. Natl. Cancer Inst.*, **95**(21), pp. 1608–1615, [PubMed Abstract].
9. Hauptmann, M., Lubin, J. H., Stewart, P. A., Hayes, R. B., and Blair, A. (2004). Mortality from solid cancers among workers in formaldehyde industries. *Am. J. Epidemiol.*, **159**(12), pp. 1117–1130, [PubMed Abstract].
10. Graves, A. B., Rosner, D., Echeverria, D., Mortimer, J. A., and Larson, E. B. (1998). Occupational exposures to solvents and aluminium and estimated risk of Alzheimer's disease. *Occup. Environ. Med.*, **55**, pp. 627–633, [PMC free article].
11. Gun, R. T., Korten, A. E., Jorm, A. F., et al. (1997). Occupational risk factors for Alzheimer disease: a case-control study. *Alz. Dis. Assoc. Dis.*, **11**, pp. 21–27.
12. Salib, E. (2000). Risk factors in clinically diagnosed Alzheimer's disease: a retrospective hospital-based case control study in Warrington. *Aging Ment. Health*, **4**, pp. 259–267.
13. Priest, N. D. (2004). The biological behaviour and bioavailability of aluminium in man, with special reference to studies employing aluminium-26 as a tracer: review and study update. *J. Environ. Monitor*, **6**, pp. 375–403.
14. Nday, C. M., Drever, B. D., Salifoglou, T., and Platt, B. (2010). Aluminium interferes with hippocampal calcium signaling in a species-specific manner. *J. Inorg. Biochem.*, **104**, pp. 919–927.
15. Jankowska, A., Madziar, B., Tomaszewicz, M., and Szutowicz, A. (2000). Acute and chronic effects of aluminum on acetyl-CoA and acetylcholine metabolism in differentiated and nondifferentiated SN56 cholinergic cells. *J. Neurosci. Res.*, **62**, pp. 615–622.

16. Letzel, S., Lang, C. J. G., Schaller, K. H., et al. (2000). Longitudinal study of neurotoxicity with occupational exposure to aluminium dust. *Neurology*, **54**, pp. 997–1000.

17. Zschocke, S. and Hansen, H. C. (2012). *Klinische Elektroenzephalographie*. Springer, Heidelberg.

18. Bhattacharjee, S., Zhao, Y., Hill, J. M., et al. (2013). Selective accumulation of aluminum in cerebral arteries in Alzheimer's disease (AD). *J. Inorg. Biochem.*, **126**, pp. 35–37, [PMC free article].

19. Klatzo, I., Wisniewski, H., and Streicher, E. (1965). Experimental production of neurofibrillary degeneration I. Light microscopic observations. *J. Neuropathol. Exp. Neurol.*, **24**, pp. 187–199.

20. Katsetos, C. D., Savory, J., Herman, M. M., et al. (1990). Neuronal cytoskeletal lesions induced in the CNS by intraventricular and intravenous aluminium maltol in rabbits. *Neuropathol. Appl. Neurobiol.*, **16**, pp. 511–528.

21. Zhang, Q. L., Jia, L., Jiao, X., et al. (2012). APP/PS1 transgenic mice treated with aluminum: an update of Alzheimer's disease model. *Int. J. Immunopathol. Pharmacol.*, **25**, pp. 49–58.

22. Ulusoy, H. B., Sonmez, M. F., Kilic, E., et al. (2015). Intraperitoneal administration of low dose aluminium in the rat: how good is It to produce a model for Alzheimer disease. *Arch. Ital. Biol.*, **153**, pp. 266–278.

23. Akiyama, H., Hosokawa, M., Kametani, F., et al. (2012). Long-term oral intake of aluminium or zinc does not accelerate Alzheimer pathology in AbetaPP and AbetaPP/tau transgenic mice. *Neuropathology*, **32**, pp. 390–397.

24. Mannello, F., Tonti, G. A., Medda, V., Simone, P., Darbre, P. D. (2011). Analysis of aluminium content and iron homeostasis in nipple aspirate fluids from healthy women and breast cancer-affected patients. *J. Appl. Toxicol.*, **31**, pp. 262–269.

25. Millos, J., Costas-Rodriguez, M., Lavilla, I., and Bendicho, C. (2009). Multiple small volume microwave-assisted digestions using conventional equipment for multielemental analysis of human breast biopsies by inductively coupled plasma optical emission spectrometry. *Talanta*, **77**, pp. 1490–1496.

26. Exley, C., Charles, L. M., Barr, L., Martin, C., Polwart, A., and Darbre, P. D. (2007). Aluminium in human breast tissue. *J. Inorg. Biochem.*, **101**, pp. 1344–1346.

27. Ng, K. H., Bradley, D. A., and Looi, L. M. (1997). Elevated trace element concentrations in malignant breast tissues. *Br. J. Radiol.*, 70, pp. 375–382.

28. Romanowicz-Makowska, H., Forma, E., Brys, M., Krajewska, W. M., and Smolarz, B. (2011). Concentration of cadmium, nickel and aluminium in female breast cancer. *Pol. J. Pathol.*, **62**, pp. 257–261.

29. Mulay, I. L., Roy, R., Knox, B. E., Suhr, N. H., and Delaney, W. E. (1971). Trace-metal analysis of cancerous and noncancerous human tissues. *J. Natl. Cancer Inst.*, **47**, pp. 1–13.

30. Mandriota, S. J., Tenan, M., Ferrari, P., and Sappino, A. P. (2016). Aluminium chloride promotes tumorigenesis and metastasis in normal murine mammary gland epithelial cells. *Int. J. Cancer*, **139**(12), pp. 2781–2790

31. http://www.salute.gov.it/imgs/C_17_pubblicazioni_2608_allegato.pdf.

32. Han, S., Lemire, J., Appanna, V. P., Auger, C., Castonguay, Z., and Appanna, V. D. (2013). How aluminum, an intracellular ROS generator promotes hepatic and neurological diseases: the metabolic tale. *Cell Biol. Toxicol.*, **29**(2), pp. 75–84.

33. Kawahara, M. and Kato-Negishi, M. (2011). Link between aluminum and the pathogenesis of Alzheimer's disease: the integration of the aluminum and amyloid cascade hypotheses. *Int. J. Alzheimers Dis.*, **17**, p. 276393.

34. Lukiw, W. J. and Pogue, A. I. (2007). Induction of specific micro RNA (miRNA) species by ROS-generating metal sulfates in primary human brain cells. *J. Inorg. Biochem.*, **101**(9), pp. 1265–1269.

35. Wu, Z., Du, Y., Xue, H., Wu, Y., and Zhou, B. (2012). Aluminum induces neurodegeneration and its toxicity arises from increased iron accumulation and reactive oxygen species (ROS) production. *Neurobiol. Aging*, **33**(1), pp. 199.e1–199.e12.

36. Kumar, V., Bal, A., and Gill, K. D. (2009). Aluminium-induced oxidative DNA damage recognition and cell-cycle disruption in different regions of rat brain. *Toxicology*, **264**(3), pp. 137–144.

37. Vanduyn, N., Settivari, R., Levora, J., Zhou, S., Unrine, J., and Nass, R. (2013). The metal transporter SMF-3/DMT-1 mediates aluminum-induced dopamine neuron degeneration. *J. Neurochem.*, **124**(1), pp. 147–157.

38. Spěváčkova, V., Kratzer, K., Čejchanová, M., and Beneš, B. (1997). Determination of some metals in biological samples for monitoring purposes. *Cent. Eur. J. Public Health*, **5**(4), pp. 177–179.

39. Bolann, B. J., Rahil-Khazen, R., Henriksen, H., Isrenn, R., and Ulvik, R. J. (2007). Evaluation of methods for trace-element determination with emphasis on their usability in the clinical routine laboratory. *Scand. J. Clin. Lab. Invest.*, **67**(4), pp. 353–366.
40. Rosin, A. (2009). The long-term consequences of exposure to lead. *Isr. Med. Assoc. J.*, **11**(11), pp. 689–694.
41. Martin, B. L. (1999). Development of a scale for the comparison of metals in enzyme action. *J. Inorg. Biochem.*, **75**(4), pp. 245–254.
42. Tomljenovic, L. (2011). Aluminum and Alzheimer's disease: after a century of controversy, is there a plausible link? *J. Alzheimers Dis.*, **23**(4), pp. 567–598.
43. McLachlan, D. R. C., Dalton, A. J., Kruck, T. P. A., et al. (1991). Intramuscular desferrioxamine in patients with Alzheimer's disease. *Lancet*, **337**(8753), pp. 1304–1308.
44. Bohrer, D., Schmidt, M., Marques, R. C., et al. (2014). Distribution of aluminum in hair of Brazilian infants and correlation to aluminum-adjuvanted vaccine exposure. *Clin. Chim. Acta*, **428**, pp. 9–13.
45. Bohrer, D., Dessuy, M. B., Kaizer, R., et al. (2008). Tissue digestion for aluminum determination in experimental animal studies. *Anal. Biochem.*, **377**(2), pp. 120–127.
46. Ivanenko, N. B., Ivanenko, A. A., Solovyev, N. D., Zeimal, A. E., Navolotskii, D. V., and Drobyshev, E. J. (2013). Biomonitoring of 20 trace elements in blood and urine of occupationally exposed workers by sector field inductively coupled plasma mass spectrometry. *Talanta*, **116**, pp. 764–769.
47. Exley, C., Ahmed, U., Polwart, A., and Bloor, R. N. (2007). Elevated urinary aluminium in current and past users of illicit heroin. *Addict. Biol.*, **12**(2), pp. 197–199.
48. Sandberg-Wollheim, M. and Olsson, T. (2013). Cerebrospinal fluid oligoclonal bands are important in the diagnosis of multiple sclerosis, unreasonably downplayed by the McDonald criteria 2010: yes. *Mult. Scler.*, **19**(6), pp. 714–716.
49. Wasi, S., Tabrez, S., and Ahmad, M. (2013). Toxicological effects of major environmental pollutants: an overview. *Environ. Monit. Assess.*, **185**(3), pp. 2585–2593.
50. Gura, K. M. (2010). Aluminum contamination in products used in parenteral nutrition: has anything changed? *Nutrition*, **26**(6), pp. 585–594.

51. Ganz, T. (2011). Hepcidin and iron regulation, 10 years later. *Blood*, **117**(17), pp. 4425–4433.

52. Perl, D. P. and Moalem, S. (2006). Aluminum and Alzheimer's disease, a personal perspective after 25 years. *J. Alzheimers Dis.*, **9**(3), pp. 291–300.

53. Yumoto, S., Kakimi, S., Ohsaki, A., and Ishikawa, A. (2009). Demonstration of aluminum in amyloid fibers in the cores of senile plaques in the brains of patients with Alzheimer's disease. *J. Inorg. Biochem.*, **103**(11), pp. 1579–1584.

54. Ruipérez, F., Mujika, J. I., Ugalde, J. M., Exley, C., and Lopez, X. (2012). Pro-oxidant activity of aluminum: promoting the Fenton reaction by reducing Fe(III) to Fe(II). *J. Inorg. Biochem.*, **117**, pp. 118–123.

55. Percy, M. E., Kruck, T. P. A., Pogue, A. I., and Lukiw, W. J. (2011). Towards the prevention of potential aluminum toxic effects and an effective treatment for Alzheimer's disease. *J. Inorg. Biochem.*, **105**(11), pp. 1505–1512.

56. Kan, W., Chien, C., Wu, C., Su, S., Hwang, J., and Wang, H. (2010). Comparison of low-dose deferoxamine versus standard-dose deferoxamine for treatment of aluminium overload among haemodialysis patients. *Nephrol. Dial. Transplant.*, **25**(5), pp. 1604–1608.

57. Sivakumar, S., Sivasubramanian, J., and Raja, B. (2012). Aluminium induced structural, metabolic alterations and protective effects of desferrioxamine in the brain tissue of mice: an FTIR study. *Spectrochim. Acta, Part A*, **99**, pp. 252–258.

58. Shrivastava, S. (2012). Combined effect of HEDTA and selenium against aluminum induced oxidative stress in rat brain. *J. Trace Elem. Med. Biol.*, **26**(2–3), pp. 210–214.

59. Exley, C., Mamutse, G., Korchazhkina, O., et al. (2006). Elevated urinary excretion of aluminium and iron in multiple sclerosis. *Mult. Scler.*, **12**(5), pp. 533–540.

60. Fulgenzi, A., Zanella, S. G., Mariani, M. M., Vietti, D., and Ferrero, M. E. (2012). A case of multiple sclerosis improvement following removal of heavy metal intoxication. *BioMetals*, **25**(3), pp. 569–576.

61. Shaw, C. A. and Tomljenovic, L. (2013). Aluminum in the central nervous system (CNS): toxicity in humans and animals, vaccine adjuvants, and autoimmunity. *Immunol. Res.*, **56**(2–3), pp. 304–316.

62. Zhu, Y. Z., Liu, D. W., Liu, Z. Y., and Li, Y. F. (2013). Impact of aluminum exposure on the immune system: a mini review. *Environ. Toxicol. Pharmacol.*, **35**(1), pp. 82–87.

63. Exley, C. (2014). What is the risk of aluminium as a neurotoxin? *Expert Rev. Neurother.*, **14**(6), pp. 589–591.

64. Bamonti, F., Fulgenzi, A., Novembrino, C., and Ferrero, M. E. (2011). Metal chelation therapy in rheumathoid arthritis: a case report. Successful management of rheumathoid arthritis by metal chelation therapy. *BioMetals*, **24**(6), pp. 1093–1098.

65. Corsello, S., Fulgenzi, A., Vietti, D., and Ferrero, M. E. (2009). The usefulness of chelation therapy for the remission of symptoms caused by previous treatment with mercury-containing pharmaceuticals: a case report. *Cases J.*, **2**(11), 199, https://casesjournal.biomedcentral.com/articles/10.1186/1757-1626-2-199.

66. https://www.supremecourt.gov/opinions/10pdf/09-152.pdf.

67. Gatti, A. and Montanari, S. (2017). New quality-control investigations on vaccines: micro- and nanocontamination. *Int. J. Vaccines Vaccin.*, **4**(1), p.00072, https://medcraveonline.com/ijvv/new-quality-control-investigations-on-vaccines-micro--and-nanocontamination.html.

68. Lavezzi, A. M., et al. (2015). Sudden infant death with area postrema lesion likely due to wrong use of insecticide. *Pediatrics*, **136**(4), pp. 1–7.

Chapter 7

How Babies Can Be Polluted

We have already said long enough about how modern man is polluting the world with a strength and an effectiveness never seen in the past.

Many of the pollutants are 'eternal', meaning that nature is not capable of transforming them into something less aggressive, and many take a long time to make their toxicity manifest. Their constant accumulation is objectively becoming a debt which our generation unloads on the next and the next will find such a huge account to settle that it will never be able to cope with it.

But without having to wait for the children to grow up and take the place in the society of those who run it today, the current pollution we are causing starts to hit them already before they are born.

7.1 Male Fertility, Burning Semen Disease and Endometriosis

For years we have been analysing the sperm of subjects exposed to pollution from inorganic micro- and nanodust, starting with soldiers who, from a certain point of view, are an excellent object of study, given that they breathe and ingest large quantities of particles in a relatively short time. In that sperm there are thoroughly undue

Advances in Nanopathology: From Vaccines to Food
Antonietta Morena Gatti and Stefano Montanari

ISBN 978-981-4877-29-9 (Hardcover), 978-1-003-05622-5 (eBook)
www.jennystanford.com

presences of the particles object of our interest. Figure 7.1 shows white lead particles close to a spermatozoon (inside red inset) of a contaminated soldier.

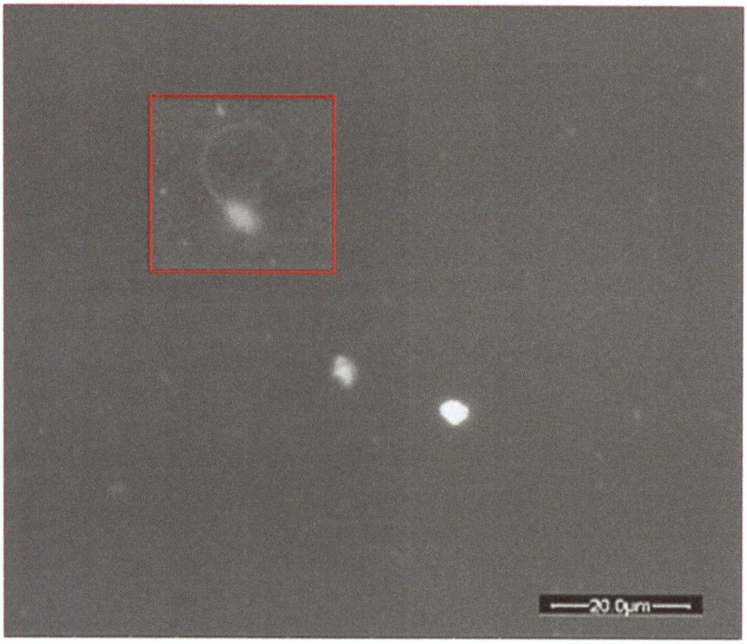

Figure 7.1 Contaminated seminal fluid.

The first symptom, although not always present, signaling those presences is a burning feeling in the penis during urination and during ejaculation. Moreover, without this being surprising, even in the sperm those particles behave according to what they are: foreign bodies. The spermatozoa count of persons exposed to a contamination decreases dramatically and so does their mobility, thereby making the male much less capable of procreation. We add that several years ago, finding ourselves facing the case of a soldier who wanted to father a child despite being in those conditions, we resorted to a 'cleaning' of the seminal fluid and artificial insemination, with the result of his wife giving birth to a pair of perfectly healthy twins.

But the most serious and painful consequences affect the female partner. We have no data available as a result of our research, but it is absolutely probable that, as happens in the blood plasma, also in the seminal fluid particles can modify the proteins, thereby making them intolerable for the epithelial tissue lining the vaginal canal. What we are being reported for years and which is becoming an increasingly widespread phenomenon is the occurrence of painful coituses, following which, if the coitus is not protected by a condom, painful, bleeding and both pharmacologically and surgically intractable ulcers are formed in the vaginal canal. This condition is called burning semen disease.

Another phenomenon which we often observe in women suffering from this pathology is the onset of endometriosis. We do not have enough data in this regard and we simply report the coincidence.

7.2 Particles from Mother to Foetus

For over 20 years we have been dealing with war pollution, and the phenomena which occur in war occur in military shooting ranges as well.

Working in the Salto di Quirra (Sardinia, Italy) shooting range on the Italian island Sardinia, we came across cattle which were brought down because they could no longer give birth and severely malformed lambs which almost always died as soon as they were born (Fig. 7.2). In all the cases of lambs we had the opportunity to analyse, their internal organs contained large quantities of particles foreign to living organisms and compatible with what is produced by explosions of armaments. Being animals born a few minutes before when not stillborn, it is evident that those particles embedded in the tissues must have been present when the foetus was inside the mother's womb. Therefore, their origin could only be from the mother and, in the mother, from what she had eaten and breathed: grass and air, respectively, polluted by the explosions.

It may be interesting to note that in some of those lambs the *linea alba*, that is, the aponeurotic structure located on the middle portion of the abdomen, had not formed. In this condition, the lamb's abdomen opened at the time of birth and the viscera were expelled. Embryological problems affecting the midline of the body, as is the position of the *linea alba*, is something which, in our experience, we have found in some children of soldiers (cleft palate and spina bifida). We are unable to provide embryological explanations, since this is not the field for which we are competent, and we limit ourselves to reporting what we have ascertained.

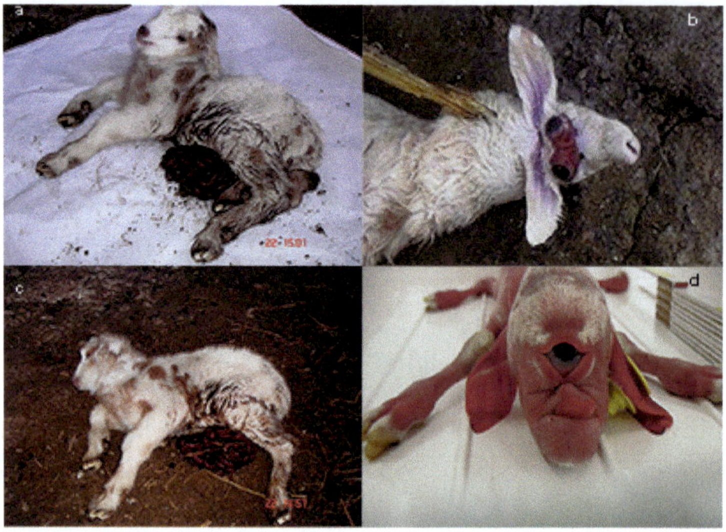

Figure 7.2 Corpses of malformed lambs from the Sardinian shooting range of Salto di Quirra (Sardinia, Italy).

Another fact which we come across with increasing frequency is the number of miscarriages within the third month of pregnancy. It is not uncommon to observe that after two or three such events, the baby who is born alive is perfectly healthy. We attribute the fact to the action of the foetuses which act as a filter, freeing the mother from the presence of inorganic particles. In this way, the embryo is unable to complete its formation but, on the other hand, leaves a clean environment for an upcoming pregnancy (Fig. 7.3).

In short, it is evident that the particles pass from mother to foetus through the placental barrier and what happens in animals happens in humans. And that's what we found when we dealt with children born with cancer. We have already described several cases of children we studied who were born already ill with cancer in our book *Nanotoxicology and Particle Toxicology* (Academic Press, 2015). We have added the case we came across of a baby born with yolk sac cancer (see Chapter 2). While all the other children born with cancer which we have analysed have died, this was operated on early and to date, after more than five years, is in good health.

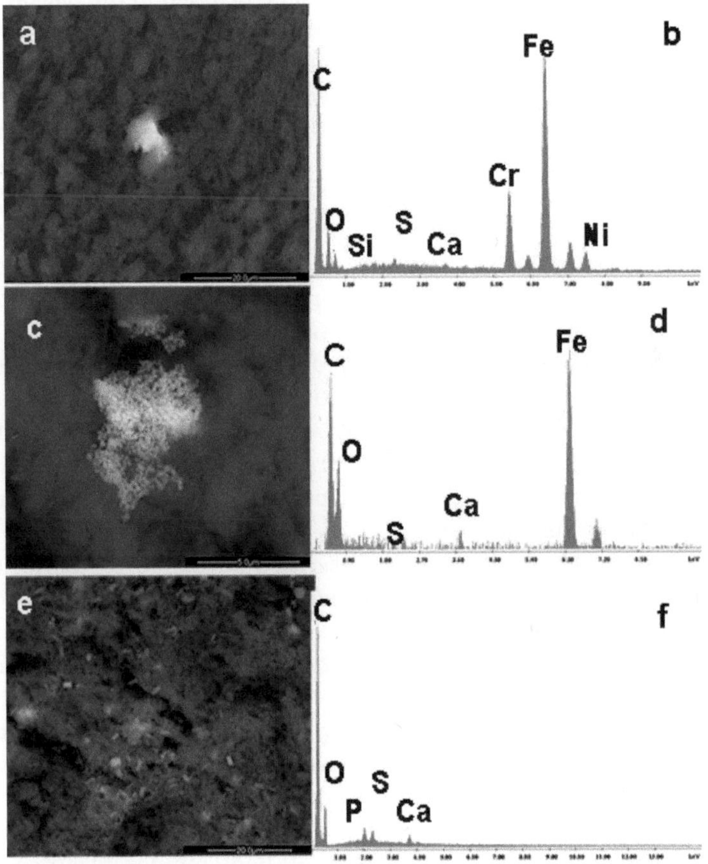

Figure 7.3 Miscarriage at a polluted site. As often happens, the tissues of aborted foetuses contain inorganic particles. In general, those particles reach the foetus through the mother's blood and derive from pollution which can be environmental or derived from food or from drugs taken during pregnancy. In this case, the particles containing a large component of chromium or steel (iron, chromium and nickel) undoubtedly come from external sources. For a better understanding, it should be borne in mind that the case comes from a small town where a large steel mill exists. The calcium- and phosphorus-based particles could have an origin within the mother's body or, albeit, in our opinion, with very little probability, within the foetus's. Their parallelepiped shape is noteworthy. Spherical iron nanoparticles are characteristic of formations within the organism (*siderosis*), and for those shown in the picture the origin is unquestionably within the organism.

7.3 Drugs Administered during Pregnancy

It is not at all uncommon that the leaflets included in the packaging of a drug warn that product is contraindicated during pregnancy or that, in any case, it must be administered only in events of real need and inability to act in any other way. Given the enormous difference between individuals and the haste with which drugs too often go into distribution, it is customers who act as guinea pigs and certain consequences are found only after years of use and, of course, not affecting all subjects. Indeed, often undue effects occur only on a relatively small fraction of those who take the drug, and it is not uncommon that, if the adverse phenomena are not excessively conspicuous and numerous, they pass over in silence.

Perhaps many remember *thalidomide*, a drug which was sold in the fifties and sixties as a sedative, anti-emetic and hypnotic, aimed especially at pregnant women. It was a drug which, according to what was presented, had an extremely favourable risk–benefit balance compared to *barbiturates* and other drugs available at the time for the same purpose.

It was only after years that it was impossible to deny how women treated with thalidomide gave birth to children with severe alterations in the development of the limbs, that is, *amelia* (absence of the limbs) or various degrees of *focomelia* (reduction of the long bones of the limbs).

The risky drugs during pregnancy are very numerous, and often they are very common medications which can be bought even over the counter and without a prescription. Antibiotics, pain relievers, psychotropic drugs and medications to lower the body temperature in the case of (almost always beneficial) body temperature rise are only a few categories of those medications.

It is not in the purposes of this book to deal in depth with that subject. We just want to mention what is strictly part of our skills and what is unequivocal from our analyses.

The habit of giving vaccines to pregnant women is becoming more and more widespread and is often recommended by media and doctors themselves. That a vaccine can immunise a foetus is doubtful to say the least. That all the vaccines we have analysed are polluted by micro- and nanoparticles which are incompatible with the body is indisputable, and the body of an embryo is small and delicate. That manufacturers warn about the opportunity to take vaccines or, at least, some of them, during pregnancy is easily a fact which anyone who takes the trouble to read the published warnings can see. So, regardless of personal beliefs which often have nothing scientific and the enormous interests which influence the vaccine business, an invitation to prudence seems reasonable to us. It would be very sad that, for vaccines as for what happened to a very long list of medicaments, something unpleasant be noticed when it is too late.

7.4 Drugs Immediately after Birth

The injection of *vitamin K* a few minutes after birth belongs to the protocol of many hospitals.

The obvious fact must be considered that the deficiency of that vitamin is rare, that it is only possible to find it in cases of particular problems related to blood clotting and, therefore, in the overwhelming majority of cases that administration is completely pointless.

The lack of vitamin K can occur in the first 24 hours of life and almost exclusively in children born to mothers who take drugs which inhibit the production of vitamin K: anti-convulsants like carbamazepine, phenytoin and barbiturates; some antibiotics; and vitamin K antagonists like *coumarin* and *warfarin*, drugs whose administration to young and active people such as, among others, pregnant women should be avoided as far as possible. Any pharmacologist knows that that type of problem is not preventable with the administration of vitamin K to the newborn, but only by supplementing that vitamin to the mother in the days preceding the birth.

Much less severe forms related to the deficiency of that vitamin can occur after a few weeks or between two weeks and six months in very serious form in babies with biliary tract problems. Cases like these are rare indeed, and it is hard to presume that a single dose of vitamin administered a few minutes after birth can retain its activity after months.

One might think that, even if it is of at least little use, that injection does not cause problems. Analysing the drug, however, we found the presence of pollutants in the form of solid inorganic particles, and since the administration takes place in subjects which weigh very little, that dose represents a high quantity in terms of proportion (Fig. 7.4).

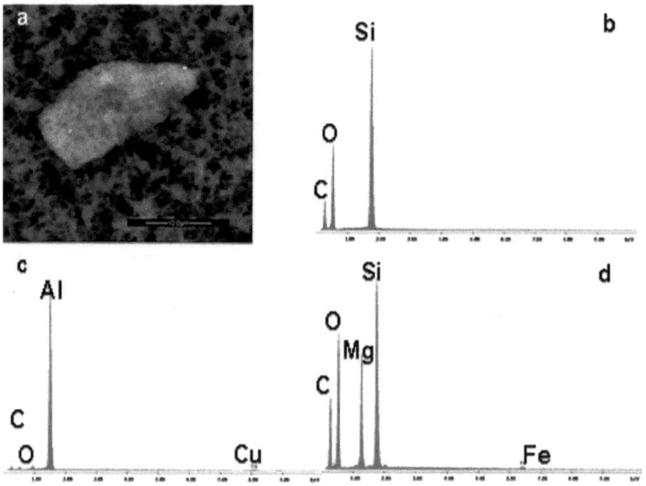

(a)

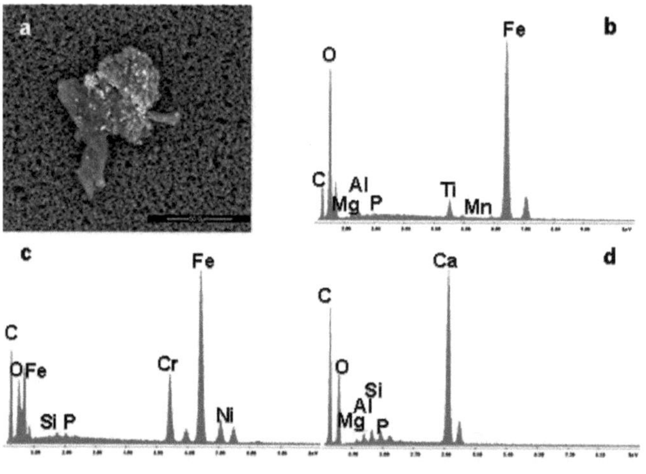

(b)

Figure 7.4 Contamination of vitamin K. The protocol of many neonatology departments requires that an injection of vitamin K be made as soon as the baby is born. Apart from any discussion about the usefulness of this administration done without carrying out any investigation showing a deficiency of that vitamin, it is worth noting the presence of polluting particles as we found in a vial of the drug (Konakion by Roche). In addition to iron-based particles, including steel ones, particles with a composition of calcium, silicon and magnesium have been found, which, without being able to be certain since it is not possible to inspect the production laboratory, appear to be common environmental dust.

A simple balance between the actually achievable benefit and the potential risk run would recommend avoiding that injection unless there is a proven indication.

In a breastfeeding woman, the particles inhaled, ingested or anyway administered can enter the lactiferous ducts and consequently end up in breast milk and be ingested by the baby. Said in parentheses, it may be interesting to investigate whether those undue presences may have any function in inducing breast cancer.

In many countries, with significant mutual differences, by law or by habit or because of personal convictions, a different number and variety of vaccines are administered to newborns. It is not our intention to debate here the possibility of immunising a newborn baby. We only want to underline how a newborn's microbiota is not able to easily tolerate those drugs containing, in addition to the active principle and as already mentioned, a long series of substances not always indicated in full by the manufacturer and not always safe (antibiotics, formaldehyde, preservatives, emulsifying agents, human and animal DNA, aluminium, etc.) and a far from indifferent quantity of pollutants. It is necessary to add that different substances (e.g. mercury) can be present in concentrations below the legal limits (legal and biological are different concepts) and, therefore, are not reported as if they were not existent. In the event of an allergy, however, even a minimal amount of substance can be harmful, even to the point of death (see, for example, the very small amount of poison injected by a bee sting in allergic adults). It is clear that it is not possible to know whether a child born a few weeks ago is allergic to certain substances, nor moreover, are checks carried out.

As a matter of fact, vaccinations to children are practiced blindly without any prior control regarding the subject's ability to tolerate substances both individually and mixed together. We also add that, in our personal experience, almost every day we come across a worrying and increasing number of children clearly damaged by vaccines. These are perfectly healthy and active children who, in the space of a few days or, sometimes, a few hours from the moment of vaccination, lose a large part of their intellectual faculties and of their ability to react to external stimuli. We believe that the stubborn attempt to deny very evident facts is not only contrary to science but to morality itself.

Furthermore, children are a favourite target of drug makers. The alarming abuse of psychotropic drugs which started in the United States is taking hold all over the world. Regardless of the inevitable toxicity of these drugs and their long-term consequences, the question we ask ourselves is whether psychotropic drugs are aimed at an eventual recovery or are not, rather, a kind of straitjacket made for children because they do not cause too much trouble. And we also wonder if those who are treated pharmacologically are always really pathologies.

Now, there are antibiotics liberally administered for small affections, not infrequently combined with immuno-suppressants such as *glucocorticoid* drugs (e.g. *dexamethasone* and *prednisolone*) and even prescribed for viral diseases against which, obviously, antibiotics have no activity. Needless to say, these abuses destroy the microbiota and induce antibiotic resistance which could become dangerous if those antibiotics become truly indispensable.

But the attacks they suffer from very common medicaments often obtainable without a prescription are much more usual.

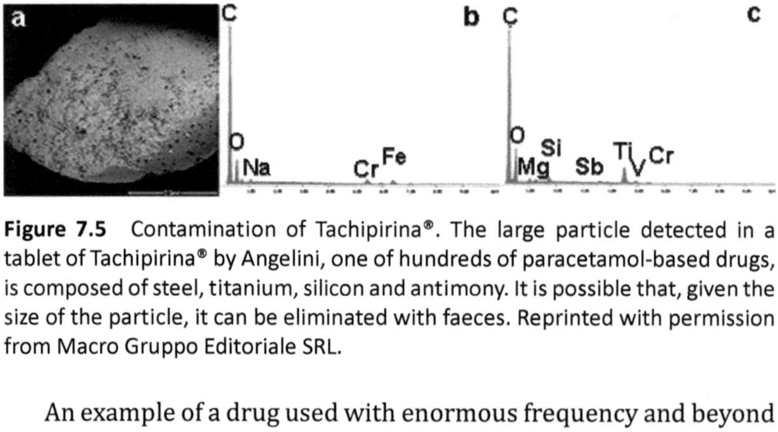

Figure 7.5 Contamination of Tachipirina®. The large particle detected in a tablet of Tachipirina® by Angelini, one of hundreds of paracetamol-based drugs, is composed of steel, titanium, silicon and antimony. It is possible that, given the size of the particle, it can be eliminated with faeces. Reprinted with permission from Macro Gruppo Editoriale SRL.

An example of a drug used with enormous frequency and beyond reason is *paracetamol* (see also Chapter 5), an active ingredient found in hundreds of different pharmaceutical forms and present in almost all homes (Fig. 7.5). What is constantly ignored is that a temperature rise is the body's first and most effective form of defense against attacks by pathogens. A higher-than-normal temperature favours the actions of the immune system and, at the same time, weakens the viruses and bacteria which are attacking. So, lowering the temperature promotes disease. A further abuse of this drug is the administration which is sometimes prescribed before the injection of a vaccine in order to avoid that the febrile reaction is detectable [1]. But, on top of all that, even those drugs can be polluted.

Finally, the food which is given to children can be polluted exactly like what any adult eats (Fig. 7.6). In the course of our research we have analysed some samples of industrial food produced exclusively for children, even when they are in their weaning phase, finding the presence of polluting particles (see Chapter 5).

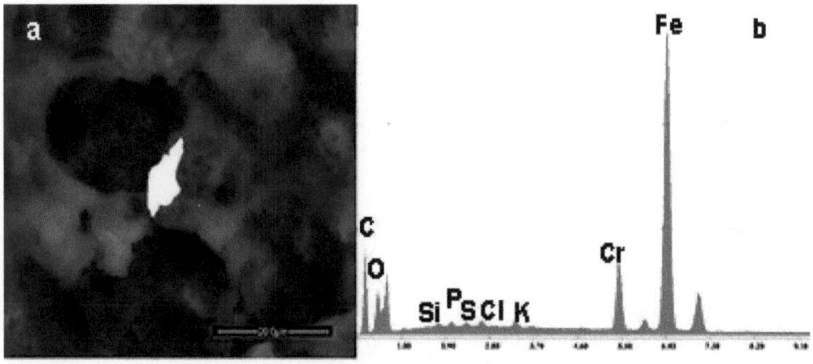

Figure 7.6 Homogenised baby food. Our analysis of homogenised rabbit meat showed the presence of steel particles. Their presence may be due to the blades being worn during the mincing process.

In this, as in almost all cases, it seems that nobody, laws and rules in the first place, deals with and worries about those presences. Thus, no adequate checks are made, and in general perception, it is as if the fact did not exist at all.

Regardless of any moral consideration, today's children are destined to be the men of tomorrow. It is clear that if the world is inhabited by a generation of sick people, the future will not be particularly bright.

Reference

1. Montanari, S. and Gatti, A. (2019). *Tachipirina®, Paracetamolo e altri Farmaci per Abbassare la Febbre: Sì o no?* Macro Edizioni, p. 96.

Chapter 8

The Future

Like any being which populates the planet, man also evolves, that is, he constantly changes his relationships with the outside world. It is a very slow process which takes many generations, but it happens constantly. This has made it possible to coexist with an unknown but enormous number of bacteria and viruses, but this will not be the case with the dust we deal with. The illusion that man can become resistant to them and that their presence in the organism becomes harmless is equivalent to thinking that one can become resistant to a bullet which crosses the heart.

So far, we have seen what the current situation is. But it belongs to human nature that we are curious about what the future has in store.

As is obvious, when trying to predict what is going to happen one must accept the existence of a margin of error, to reduce which it is necessary not to neglect anything of the notions which are available. So, let's make a very brief summary.

As far as we have been able to see after some decades of research and thousands of cases studied involving human and animal tissues, the environment, food, drugs and a variety of other products, particulate matter is becoming more and more present in our world with no possibility of decline. Man's growing ability to use new technical and industrial very-high-temperature processes – temperatures which are definitely higher than those used in the

Advances in Nanopathology: From Vaccines to Food
Antonietta Morena Gatti and Stefano Montanari

ISBN 978-981-4877-29-9 (Hardcover), 978-1-003-05622-5 (eBook)
www.jennystanford.com

past – involves the fact that the particles produced as a side effect are much finer and, as a first consequence though certainly not the sole, are much more capable of penetrating biological tissues. As we have briefly described, particles of natural and incidental origin as an unwanted product of many technologies; particles created specifically in specialised laboratories to meet the needs of nanotechnologies, are increasingly being added to the environment and, as an obvious consequence, to our body.

No matter what their origin and purpose are, tissues perceive them for what they are: foreign bodies. And their set of reactions can't be other than the one foreign bodies trigger. One of the aggravating circumstances is that fine and ultrafine particles can enter cell nuclei and interfere with the DNA in a way and with consequences which we are not yet fully able to predict. Another problem is that those particles can negotiate virtually any physiological barriers, including the brain and the placental blood circulation.

Regardless of the solid, inorganic particles produced by nature, which are by far the least aggressive, for the most part those found in the environment derive from processes which are, one way or another, related to economic activities and, ultimately, to money.

The first consequence is that the study of particulate matter's behaviour either in the environment or in the living organisms is biased by economic interest: anything but a novelty. It is enough to read what was written not much long ago by scientists about tobacco, asbestos, tetraethyl lead, chlorofluorocarbons and many other noxious substances on whose toxicity there are no discussions today to realise the fact. Unquestionably harmful today, yet, not a few years ago, those products were considered the most harmless things there were in the world and anyone who dared to argue otherwise was branded as an enemy of science and progress. So, as expected, though with a very slightly waning vivacity, particles also have their defendants according to whom they are harmless.

As for the future, much, perhaps everything, will depend on how much the huge and various financial interests linked to the particles will affect the laws and the way of representing reality.

It may appear bizarre, but in many cases the scientific knowledge acquired is in stark contrast to what is put into practice. The possible examples are very numerous. Among the many possible, there is that of foreign bodies inside the tissues. It is widely known, and for a very long time widely accepted without any objection, that these cause the formation of inflammatory processes and that those processes, becoming chronic as is the case with indestructible inductors like so many inorganic particles, cause the transformation of previously healthy tissues into cancerous ones. Yet, when those very same particles are born out of processes involving major rounds of money, everything is forgotten or, worse, denied.

Their presence as pollutants in various drugs, first of all vaccines, is normally judged as irrelevant. Notoriously non-biodegradable inorganic particles are regularly used as excipients in drugs and as additives in food, and no one seems to pose problems in this regard, as if the body made differences between unwanted particles, particles which come in handy for someone and particles which, whatever the reason, are ignored. As is the case for vaccines with regards to whose particle pollution there can be no doubt, systems such as particulate filters for diesel engines are made mandatory with the consequent release into the atmosphere of tiny particles which would otherwise have remained enclosed in carbonaceous formations, much coarser and, therefore, much less aggressive for health. Another example is the one concerning aluminium. For many years its toxicity has been widely known, especially at the level of the central nervous system, and as a possible carcinogen, so much so that the Italian Ministry of Health writes verbatim, 'The main suspect – to be verified – on an association between aluminium and increased tumor risk in the human being concern the possible association between breast cancer and the use of deodorants containing aluminium requires that, when there are doubts about the tolerability of a substance, its use is suspended until certainties have been reached' [1, 2].

Still, aluminium is regularly added as adjuvant to vaccines which are injected even in premature babies and pregnant women.

We could go on for several pages, but we believe the concept is clear. And from the concept we can only draw the conclusion that, if what we want is a future which allows an acceptably healthy life, we can do nothing but behave according to what real, coldly neutral, scientific knowledge imposes. Ultimately, the solution lies in honesty, in any way one wants to consider it.

What *Homo sapiens* must necessarily realise is that nature behaves according to unchangeable laws and that she does not care about the interests, whims, pretensions, illusions and laziness of man, that is, of an animal which the world can spare without problems. Indeed, if the planet should do without man, many problems would simply become non-existent.

Unfortunately, in the last few decades we have polluted the planet and, consequently, ourselves, much more than we have done in thousands of centuries and not a little of that pollution is without possible return. At least, not in a short time.

The only thing we can do, abandoning the naive illusion that the planet is endowed with a sort of rapid homeostasis, is to stop and review our whole lifestyle. Of course, it is not easy, since bad habits are the easiest to take and the most difficult to remove, but there is no other possibility, because with nature there is no room for negotiation.

Contrary to what is not rarely heard objecting, this does not imply a 'return to the caves', even if, from a merely objective point of view, however unacceptable for us authors first, a world without fire and without technologies would be the most effective countermeasure against the current situation. This implies the uncompromising use of scientific knowledge and the development of far more advanced technologies than those, all things considered, rough and largely incomplete, which we use today. Therefore, it would be a turn towards the application of the notions which we have reached over centuries of science.

A concept as fundamental as it has always been known is that of prevention. 'Prevention is better than cure' and 'better be safe than sorry' are part of popular wisdom.

Prevention in strict terms is that which prevents the occurrence of a harmful situation. Staying in the field of health, very trivially, countermeasures are put in place to avoid getting sick. For those who are fond of classifications, this is *primary prevention*. In practical terms, this is by far the most effective type of prevention and by far the least expensive. But it is precisely the fact of having these two characteristics which makes it much less practiced than it should reasonably be. The cash turnover which the disease ensures is enormous, and those involved in the business do not see favourably something which can in any way slow down their activity. Hence, all the absurdities condemned by science but widely practiced which have just been, and only partially, mentioned.

The step which follows in a direction surely more appreciated by those who make health their business is that of the so-called *secondary prevention*. This is nothing more than the early detection of diseases or a warning which one may be at risk of contracting a disease, which means periodically undergoing a checkup, which, in turn, entails expenses which may not be trivial. We would not want to be misunderstood: Diagnosing a disease onset means increasing the chances of recovery considerably. Predicting the onset of a not-yet-existing pathological condition can even seem miraculous. But the obvious question is, To what diseases will we target our early diagnosis? The diseases we know are several thousand (only the diseases which we call orphans, that is, without a therapy, have been registered in the order of magnitude of about 10,000), and there is no diagnostic method capable of diagnosing them early if not in a very minimal proportion. And even when the suspected diseases are very few when not a single one, it is not so rare that the diagnostic assessment does not enjoy an acceptable degree of accuracy. It is the personal experience of the two of us who write these notes to have come across patients diagnosed with a disease (e.g. a cardiovascular pathology) checked and declared free of immediate problems, just to die after a few days. In the same way, but on the contrary, it is our experience that of having known patients declared to be either at imminent danger of life or judged on the path of aggravation of an already diagnosed disease or at serious risk to contract it (e.g. a cancer), who lived happily for decades, almost always without a trace of the feared disease. Thus, without wanting to diminish the importance of more or less general checkups or periodic medical checks for some disease, blindly trusting them can lead to false security or lead to objectively unjustified states of anxiety. In short, with secondary prevention, we significantly recede with respect to the effects guaranteed by approaches which tend to prevent the onset of a pathology or, much more often, of a series of pathologies. There is no doubt, however, that this approach guarantees a remarkable and lasting business. This is also because to prevent a disease, drugs are often prescribed almost never taking due account of their side effects which, however, are largely, albeit with some 'shyness' and some 'modesty', declared by the producers themselves.

Then, when the disease really outbreaks, in addition to continuing with the obvious and indispensable checks, the so-called *tertiary prevention* is put in place, which, in reality, aims to but prevent an aggravation or early death, a condition, the latter, however inevitable. And then, drugs arrive on a large scale: the most profitable business of after all an objectively failed prevention.

Having said all this, it is clear that a desirable future cannot be that of a world made up of patients who undergo a therapy which can also be very effective but a future made up of healthy people. And, then, without absolutely denying the importance of secondary and tertiary, we should focus on primary prevention as a first choice.

We have mentioned how, provided we want to enjoy an acceptable future for ourselves or, at least, to offer an acceptable one to the next generation, it is essential that we make our lifestyle less impacting on the environment and, consequently, on health.

Among the many modern problems, one of growing importance is that of waste production.

We will not go back to something we have already covered, but in summary, we would like to emphasise again that the easiest waste to treat is that which is not there.

Inevitably, to produce less waste it is necessary to use less objects, which means, sadly for those who make the production and sale of goods the economic support of their lives, to buy only the objects which we really need. As we have seen, their fate when objects are no longer needed is almost never taken care of and often they are burned, with the consequence of finding them, transformed into something much more aggressive than they were in origin, in our bodies. Continuing on this path, objects must have a life which is as long as possible and which, when in the form they have acquired are not really usable anymore, can be transformed into something else. But, if we want to be more virtuous and more effective, those materials and objects must have the least possible impact on the environment and health. This is largely a matter of culture. If the users of the products, the so-called consumers (a decidedly telling word), become capable to choose the most tolerable ones by the world we live in and avoid buying the others, the consequence, not only the most obvious but also the quickest one to occur, will be that the producers will cease immediately to manufacture them, not finding a commercial outlet.

In short, much of the future depends on us.

Another very important source of pollution comes from the movements which, apart from those made for pleasure, we are constantly forced to make for many reasons.

We have seen how unsuccessful the attempt, completely out of all scientific knowledge, yet imposed by the law, is to apply illusory devices against the pollution of diesel engines.

Apart from many ways to limit the necessity to travel, from the work often possible at home, including – as is our case – conferences sometimes located in remote places, to the possibility of contacting public bodies or consultants through telematics, the most reasonable system to prevent the means of locomotion from emitting too many pollutants, and among them the particles which are the core of this book, is to make engines consume less fuel.

Very rarely, internal combustion engines have an efficiency which exceeds 30%, where efficiency is the ratio between the mechanical energy generated by the engine and the energy supplied by the fuel. Which means that, in the best conditions, over two-thirds of the energy is wasted. Therefore, rather than trying to envisage patches, it is wiser and far more convenient to make sure that the problem is as small as possible.

It is a fact that there is more than one proposal in that direction, but they are all regularly discarded in favour of the use of oil, that is, an asset which, being contained in an obviously limited quantity in the closed system of which we are part, sooner or later cannot but run out. If there was a need for further demonstration of man's intellectual myopia, here it is.

But, leaving aside global strategies which would require the involvement of large centres of political and economic power, something can be done advantageously on a smaller scale.

For some years, devices which filter the dust present in houses or in particularly critical places such as hospitals have become increasingly popular. The differences between model and model can be quite remarkable, but they all show some efficacy. Their use should be the rule in hospitals, where, due to pollution from both dust and biologics, the possibility of contracting diseases is very high for hospitalised patients.

8.1 Particle Removal from Blood

A sentence perhaps erroneously attributed to the Latin historian Sallust reads 'faber est suae quisque fortunae', which, translated, means that 'everyone is the architect' (the blacksmith, if one wants a literal translation) of their fate. Thus, it will be us, both as a whole society and according to the behaviour of each individual, who decide what the future which awaits us will be.

If what we want is a future in which we aim exclusively at health by trying first not to lose it and, if it is unfortunately lost, to recover it in the best possible way, it is inevitable that we must avoid the use of drugs which not infrequently becomes an abuse. We have already seen, in fact, how there is no drug without side effects, and it is not uncommon for those effects to be worse than the disease they should cure.

But we deal with solid, inorganic and non-degradable micro- and nanoparticles, whatever their origin, and in the more than 20 years dedicated to that topic, we have found that a large and, unfortunately, increasing quantity of pathologies derives from the interference of small dust with our body.

Therefore, it seems reasonable to us that it is indispensable to detect the pollution source in order to be able to remove the subject from it. It seems as reasonable to us to think that removing those particles from the blood could be an effective form of prevention or, in some cases, of therapy. This, at least, when the particles are still in the blood.

Several years ago, we carried out a very simple experiment in our laboratory using the few means we had available. We tried to remove the micro- and nanoparticles which were present in the blood and the result was very encouraging.

The system had the advantage of being easy to use, scarcely invasive and repeatable without contraindications. Therefore, it could be used to clean from particles the blood of those who, for whatever reason, had undergone exposure to dust. This could be applied both to acute cases, such as what happens to firefighters when they are called to put out a fire, and to cases of prolonged or chronic intoxication as happens to soldiers, to those who work in the numerous polluted factories or to the urban police continuously exposed to traffic, etc.

It is quite possible that a filter based on the knowledge of nanotechnology already acquired and that which could be developed if one focused on the problem could be designed and produced. Of course, what we have experimentally developed in our laboratory should be engineered in such a way as to be able to make available to medicine an apparatus and a filter which can be used routinely without difficulty and without particular inconvenience for the subject who undergoes the 'cleaning'. The idea, however, was not followed up due to the lack of the funds needed for the necessary engineering and careful experimentation. Still, we are waiting for an industry in the sector to decide that some effort in this direction is worthwhile.

8.2 Conclusions

But now the question is, What will the future be like?

The question has existed since man exists, and no oracle has ever had an acceptable degree of accuracy.

The possible extrapolations are infinite, and everyone is free to choose the one they like best. We can only say that today, as has often been the case in history, much of the future is in our hands. One thing is certain: the path we have taken satisfies our laziness and our being spoiled children. This is a dead end. If we want the next generation not to ask us too embarrassing questions, we will necessarily have to rethink our lifestyle and we will have to apply science for what it really is and not for what we naively want to delude ourselves that it is.

References

1. http://www.salute.gov.it/imgs/C_17_pubblicazioni_2608_allegato.pdf.
2. https://ec.europa.eu/environment/chemicals/reach/pdf/publications/final_report_pp.pdf.

Index